The Temperamental Thread

THE TEMPERAMENTAL THREAD

How Genes, Culture, Time, and Luck Make Us Who We Are

Jerome Kagan

DANA
PRESS

New York

2010

DANA
PRESS

Published by
The Dana Foundation
745 Fifth Avenue, Suite 900
New York, NY 10151

DANA is a federally registered trademark

ISBN-13: 978-1-932594-50-8

Library of Congress Cataloging-in-Publication Data
    Kagan, Jerome.
        The temperamental thread : how genes, culture, time and luck make us who we are
        / Jerome Kagan.
            p. cm.
        Includes bibliographical references and index.
        ISBN 978-1-932594-50-8 (cloth)
        1. Temperament. I. Title.
BF798.K34 2010
155.2'34—dc22
        2009044004

Cover design by Kenneth Krattenmaker
Inside design by William Stilwell

Printed in the United States of America

Credits

Contents

Illustrations

Acknowledgments

I am deeply grateful to Jane Nevins for her superb editing of the manuscript and enthusiasm for this project, to Amanda Cushman, who carried out the initial edit, and to Paula Mabee for her able typing assistance.

Foreword

Jerome Kagan's beautiful essay is about temperamental variation in behavior, its causes and consequences. It richly situates
temperament in biological and social context and illustrates the
importance for adult development of small variations that emerge
very early in life. The work featured in this essay is the product of
a career of one of America's great psychologists of the twentieth
and twenty-first centuries. Readers will be treated to a breath-
taking scope and synthesis that is unfortunately all too rare among
today's super-specialized scientists.

Kagan's work stands as the most important body of modern work
on temperament. What makes his analysis so compelling is the
extraordinary range of data and disciplines from which he draws.
This kind of blending of research across fields is not just a luxury to
behold, but increasingly a necessity to make genuine progress.

The study of temperament invites us to consider the role of
variation in human emotional response. Temperament refers to

particular types of variation that are observable from very early in life and are assumed to be at least in part heritable, which recent evidence clearly indicates is the case. And some evidence exists that at least some of these dimensions of temperament are modestly stable.

The fact of variation among people in how they respond to emotional challenges is probably the most noticeable quality of emotion. Different toddlers as well as different adults respond noticeably differently to life's slings and arrows. As Kagan's essay makes very clear, variation in temperament and in other emotional characteristics is key to understanding human personality and vulnerability to psychopathology. Why one person is likely to decompensate quickly in response to adversity while another shows resilience is in part a product of differences in temperament. Thus the study of temperament is central to many of the key questions that have fascinated philosophers and psychologists over the ages.

As Kagan shows us, variations in temperament are accompanied by variations not only in brain function, but also in patterns of peripheral biology—that is, biology below the neck. This includes the autonomic nervous system, the endocrine system and the immune system. For each of these systems, there is bidirectional communication with the brain; the brain can influence functioning in these systems, and different patterns of activity in these systems provide feedback to brain and modulate its activity. Some reports have found small but systematic differences in vulnerability to particular types of physical disorders among those with specific temperament types. Such non-random associations imply that the neural systems underlying particular temperamental types also exert some influence on peripheral biological systems to increase the vulnerability of an individual to certain types of illnesses, such as allergies. This work will help to place the mind back into biomedicine by specifically illustrating how the brain might influence the periphery in ways that are important for health.

In the Preface to William James's *The Principles of Psychology* published 120 years ago, James wrote that the brain was the immediate organ that underlies all of our mental operations and then went on to say that the whole remainder of the *Principles* was but a footnote to this single claim. While James had a strong intuition about the role of the brain in behavior, it was not until the late twentieth century that science developed tools to non-invasively interrogate the human brain and examine changes during specific mental tasks. This technological development enabled both psychologists and the lay public to more readily appreciate James's claim. Any behavioral variation must be "caused" by the brain. That is, the nearest or most immediate cause must be rooted in variation in brain function, since there is no other organ that underlies behavior. If two children differ in some temperamental characteristic, a difference in their brains must be associated with this temperamental difference. This is what we might refer to as a *proximal* cause. If it were possible to go into a person's brain and stimulate specific circuits known to be involved in a particular temperamental quality, we might transiently alter that person's temperament. And in fact some findings in the scientific literature indicate that direct stimulation of the amgydala, a key limbic site you will learn more about in the pages ahead, can provoke a transient increase in experienced fear and autonomic changes that often accompany fear. Precisely this type of study has been conducted in patients about to undergo neurosurgery who have electrodes implanted deep within their brain to measure electrical signals that might reflect epilepsy, for example. Such findings have helped establish the amygdala as a key structure in the emotional circuit, the activity of which can be said to be a proximal cause of fear.

In a very general way, given the role of the brain in all complex behavior, it can be said that for all mental operations the brain is the proximal cause. It should be apparent, though, that knowing this gives us absolutely no clue about the *distal*—or outlying— cause. Thus we might identify the key neural circuits that underlie some of the temperamental variation described in these pages, but this information says nothing about the factors that might have caused the brain to be this way in the first place. And here there are two important points to emphasize. One is that, based upon everything we know about temperament (much of it summarized in what follows), it is certainly likely that some of the variation is caused by heritable factors, and many genes—not a single gene— probably contribute to any temperamental quality. Complex behavior is much like most complex human diseases, which are affected by a large number of genes acting in concert. The second issue of great importance stems from the fact of neuroplasticity. The brain is the organ built to change in response to experience and learning. This fact allows for a very large set of influences to shape brain circuits that might be important for temperament. Thus, how a parent behaves toward his or her child literally affects the child's brain development. Rigorous studies in animals have documented that how a mother behaves toward its offspring can literally alter gene expression in the offspring, and this alteration in gene expression can then produce lasting behavioral changes. A specific example pertains directly to the types of temperament you will be introduced to in Kagan's essay. If a rat bred to be highly anxious is reared by a mother who is very nurturing, which in the rodent world is expressed as high levels of licking and grooming, then the offspring shows much reduced anxiety. Most important, the expression of some genes directly implicated in aspects of anxiety is down-regulated by the behavior of the mother. Thus, the mother's behavior induces a change in gene expression in the offspring exclusively through her behavioral interactions with her infant. Such changes in gene expression can persist for the entire duration of the lifetime of the offspring. This suggests that the proximal causes of temperament in the brain can be altered by a distal cause: experience.

A central feature of the work summarized in these pages is that certain very early signs of temperament can be objectively measured. These behavioral and physiological signs are observable within the first 4 months of life. While many parents form early impressions of their child's temperament, the temperament and personality of a parent interacts with that of the child, and some parents are less aware of these features than others. Knowing something about the early temperament of one's child can be very helpful since it would allow a parent to better prepare for how the child might behave in certain circumstances and make adjustments to encourage the best outcomes. This kind of knowledge also might be useful to teachers and caregivers by helping to match a child's temperament with the specific child care and teaching methods that would be most beneficial in promoting positive life outcomes as the child develops. While we are still some ways away from a quick and reliable assessment of a range of temperamental variation, the fact that these variations can be measured very early in life can be potentially harnessed for use by those who come in most frequent contact with the child. How we might best match a child's specific temperament with parenting, care giving and teaching practices to yield the most beneficial outcome is a question that has not yet received enough serious research attention, but is one that will follow from the work presented here. Jerome Kagan and his colleagues have shown us that some temperamental types are associated with increased vulnerability to anxiety and mood disorders, all other things being equal. This important fact invites us to consider the possibility of utilizing preventative strategies if we know a child may be at elevated risk. It will be important in the future to conduct longitudinal studies of preventative strategies in children who are temperamentally at risk.

A fascinating consideration this essay brings to mind is about temperamental variation and the division of labor in society. Readers will be treated to an engaging description of the developmental unfolding of temperament from a scientist who has conducted some of the longest and most important longitudinal studies on this topic. The ability to track development from early in the first year through adolescence and early adulthood is very precious and does not occur often. In this work we learn of extraordinarily talented individuals who as youngsters were highly socially anxious yet go on to pursue successful careers, such as in engineering or computing, that require little social interaction. Kagan shows us how the environment can shape early temperament in socially productive and rewarding ways for the individual. The many roles and occupations in our complex society require that we have a population with a very wide range of skills and dispositions. Outgoing and gregarious individuals are wonderful for certain types of occupations but probably would not make good air traffic controllers. For our world to function it is critical that we have a very diverse array of talents and temperaments. In this essay we are treated to compelling life stories of individuals at opposite ends of the spectrum in their reactivity to novelty, many of whom develop into very happy and productive adults.

What seems to matter most for life success is a good match between an individual's temperament and the environmental context in which she or he develops. The study of temperament underscores the importance of human variation and illustrates the danger of lapsing into cultural stereotypes about ideal temperamental types. There is no ideal temperament. There might be optimal matches between a temperamental type and a particular environmental context, and, when such optimal matches occur, we all benefit from them.

How immutable is temperament? A key fact about temperament is underscored repeatedly in this essay. Namely, it is multi-determined and there is no single factor that can account for its expression. Having said that, some evidence also indicates that moderate stability exists over time for at least some temperamental types. Despite this stability, change also clearly occurs, and examples of major environmental changes that precipitate alterations in temperament are described in this essay. As noted earlier, basic research in neuroscience and molecular biology provides a powerful framework for understanding how change in temperament can come about. Even for temperamental characteristics that clearly have a heritable contribution, the environment can play a major role in shaping its expression.

One of the most noteworthy insights to emerge from modern neuroscience is that of neuroplasticity: the fact that the brain is the organ built to change in response to experience. More than any other organ in our body, the brain is equipped to be transformed by experience. Indeed this capacity of the brain is what permits learning to occur. We also know that systematic training can induce specific plastic changes in the brain. For example, there are studies using modern brain imaging methods that show how musical training can induce actual structural change in the brain. In other domains, recent studies indicate that learning a complex skill such as juggling induces measurable changes in the brain. While systematic studies of training methods designed to alter or cultivate specific temperamental qualities have not been done, we do know that psychological treatments, such as cognitive behavior therapy, that produce behavioral change induce specific changes in brain function that might be associated with some change in the underlying neurobiological systems subserving particular temperamental variations.

Kagan's closing thoughts, about words and states, most concern those of us who study the mind, but should matter to everyone trying to understand emotions and temperament. His life work has led him to consider the important question of how we refer to psychological states and brain states. He has forcefully reminded us that the meaning of a construct is properly revealed by the measures that are used to operationalize it. Psychologists are permissive in their use of emotion state terms. Consider the word "fear", a word at the center of the work Kagan describes. Psychologists are permissive in their use of emotion state terms. The same word has been used to refer to the following three situations: the behavior of a rat in response to a tone that has been paired with an electric shock; the experience of infant in a study who peers down on the deep side of a visual cliff designed to simulate being of the edge of a precipitous height; and the experience of an adult waiting to learn the results of a biopsy that might reveal cancer. While each of these three instances might have something in common, it is also clear that they differ in important ways and that it is probably inappropriate to use the same word to refer to all three since it implies that they are actually the same. It will be of interest to empirically examine what, if anything, is common about the brain states among these three types of experiences, rather than assume that they reflect the same brain state. This project is one of the many that remain for the next generations of scientists to tackle. May the work of Jerome Kagan serve as inspiring example for the next generation of scholars to carefully balance breadth and depth in their pursuit of what makes us human.

—Richard J. Davidson
Laboratory for Affective Neuroscience
University of Wisconsin-Madison

1

Introduction

What Are Human Temperaments?

An attractive sixteen-year-old high school junior, Marjorie, wearing a white blouse buttoned to her neck, sits stiffly on a hard chair for a three-hour interview in the living room of her home in a middle-class Boston suburb. Her replies to the initial questions about schoolwork and hobbies are typical of teenage girls from her social class, although they are terse, spoken in a soft voice, and accompanied by restless fidgeting with face, hair, or clothes, few spontaneous smiles, and frequent bursts of eyeblinks. Humans begin to blink rapidly when they are feeling uncertain or anxious.

Marjorie tells Valerie, the interviewer, that she has a good relationship with her affectionate parents, several close friends, usually gets A's along with a few B's in her courses, and prefers the solitary hobby of tennis to team sports like soccer. She is beginning to think about the college applications she has to complete next year, and at the moment she believes that she would like to become a teacher.

However, when Valerie asks Marjorie about her worries and her moods, her answers reveal that she is not a typical adolescent.

She cannot sleep before important examinations, and sometimes vomits on evenings when she is excessively anxious about her performance the next day. She dislikes meeting strangers, feels uneasy when touched, and is worried about an imminent class trip to Washington, D.C., because she is not sure how she will feel in an unfamiliar city talking with adolescents she does not know well. Marjorie is reluctant to ride the subway from her suburb into Boston because the experience is novel; she has frequent nightmares, and often has to suppress the threatening thought that her parents might be killed in an automobile accident. Surprisingly, neither her teachers nor her friends are aware of her private apprehensions; they regard her as a conscientious, although quiet, adolescent who has no need to see a psychiatrist.

A few days earlier, Valerie had interviewed Lisa, an equally attractive sixteen-year-old high school junior from a nearby middle-class suburb who presented a dramatically different persona. Lisa, dressed in a loose-fitting sweater and a short skirt, sat on a sofa with her legs tucked up. She reported that she loves variety, enjoys visiting new places, and is president of her class and a member of the school chorale and the soccer team. She sleeps deeply, rarely has nightmares, gets excellent grades without brooding about examinations. Her answers often slid into a garrulous offering of anecdotes, accompanied by frequent smiles, bursts of laughter, a relaxed posture, and facial expressions free of eyeblinks.

No one who watched the films of the first twenty minutes of these two interviews would have difficulty recognizing that the two girls possess very different personalities, even though their environments are similar—both live with loving, two-parent families in quiet neighborhoods with excellent schools. The contrast between Marjorie and Lisa is reminiscent of the difference between the cautious, compulsive, melancholic Felix and the relaxed, impulsive, fun-loving Oscar in the popular film *The Odd Couple*. Although the differences between Felix and Oscar are unusually salient, no two people selected at random possess exactly the same personality. Human temperaments contribute to this variation, and continued research on these biological biases will remove some of the mystery surrounding each person's unique personality profile.

During the period between the two world wars, when Freud's ideas were popular, most psychologists and psychiatrists would have explained the differences between Marjorie and Lisa by speculating that experiences in their homes and with friends created the motives, emotions, and behavioral styles that differentiate the two girls. These experts might have suggested that Marjorie's mother severely criticized minor acts of disobedience or displays of anger and that Marjorie felt guilty about her vivid sexual fantasies and jealous of her more accomplished sister. These psychologists might have argued that Lisa's permissive parents allowed her to develop a conscience free of excessive guilt over envy of her accomplished brother or her sexual desires and occasional petting with her boyfriend.

From adolescence through my time as a graduate student at Yale in 1950, I accepted these explanations as obvious truths. As a teenager living in a politically liberal Jewish family in a small town in New Jersey, I remember, I argued regularly with my mother over her insistence that inborn traits were the primary determinants of a personality type. I recall writing the word "NO" in red ink on a page in a book by Francis Crick, the co-discoverer of the structure of DNA, stating that the brain's chemistry was the major determinant of the variation in human behavior. My mother's opinions, which were untouched by the "facts" that psychologists cited to support their faith in the power of experience to overcome any initial tendencies that genes might have created, sprang from her intuitions. Her conviction that people were born with emotions and habits that were preserved indefinitely, in accord with an old Spanish saying, "Nature and features last to the grave," was never swayed by any of the arguments I presented. But, of course, I failed to appreciate that my position, too, was based in part on unproven intuitions that I was using to explain my hopes, doubts, and anxious moods. I had decided that the uneasiness I felt with boys who were stronger or more attractive to girls, my occasional nightmares, and the emotionally tinged memories of stuttering as a kindergarten child were due to an overprotective mother, a dour father suffering from painful arthritis of both hips, and being the occasional target of cruel anti-Semitic taunts by a few of my classmates.

Every adolescent feels moments of tension or outright anxiety and tries to figure out the cause of these unpleasant interruptions of serene afternoons. Most have a choice among a number of villains. Some teenagers are homely, shorter or fatter than their friends, unable to get high grades even in a subject they like, clumsy on the athletic field, rejected by school cliques, severely criticized by a parent, have an alcoholic father and/or a depressed mother, live in poverty in a disorganized neighborhood, or belong to a religious or ethnic minority that a majority believes has undesirable traits. Most adolescents select the single condition, or combination of a few conditions, that they believe is the cause of their most intense moments of unhappiness, even though their private diagnosis is not always the one that research evidence would nominate as critical. Youth from economically secure families belonging to the majority ethnic and religious groups usually blame their parents for dissatisfactions with the self because they cannot think of any other reason for their angst. Youth from poor minority groups more often blame others in their society for their moments of anxiety or anger, even though they may have had parents who were as critical or rejecting as those of the middle-class youth.

I had concluded that my father's unpredictable temper, my mother's restrictiveness, and my membership in an ethnic minority that was a target of prejudice were the reasons for my doubts, and I felt certain that nothing would sway me from that belief. So what happened to change my mind after my graduate years at Yale and the decade that followed?

I first began to question my inflexible commitment to the dominating influence of nurture in 1961, when Howard Moss and I were reflecting on the personalities of seventy-one adults in their third decade who had grown up in the 1930s in southwestern Ohio. The adults were members of a longitudinal study of development conducted at the Fels Research Institute on the campus of Antioch College in the small town of Yellow Springs, midway between Columbus and Cincinnati. When I was still a young child the staff of the institute had begun observing and testing these children, from the first months of life through late adolescence. I interviewed and tested them as adults, while Howard evaluated the information that had been gathered on their childhood traits. He was unaware of their adult features; I was unaware of their childhoods.

What we discovered forced me to acknowledge the validity of my mother's intuition. A group of ten children who had been extremely timid, fearful, and shy during their first three years said during their interviews as adults that they often felt unsure, relied a great deal on their parents or, if married, their spouse, for advice, avoided risky hobbies, and were reluctant to take on difficult challenges. The four most fearful boys from this group of ten had chosen the intellectual vocations of music teacher, physicist, biologist, or psychologist, which allowed them to control the amount of unanticipated stress that might occur during the day. The three boys who had been the most fearless during their first three years selected careers that had more uncertainty, namely, high school football coach, entrepreneurial businessman, and self-employed engineer.

I was also impressed by two biological features that differentiated the very timid children from the very bold ones. As adults, the former were more likely to possess physiological measures indicating a highly reactive sympathetic nervous system, often seen in adults who are under stress and feeling anxious. The sympathetic nervous system, which lies along the spinal column, influences many bodily functions, including heart rate and blood pressure, that prepare a person to deal with a threat or to flee from it. Their second feature was a tall, thin body build, which many shared with one or both parents. I could not account for these two features by attributing them to experiences in their families. Hence, when Howard and I were writing *Birth to Maturity* (the 1962 book that summarized the project), we suggested that the differences between extreme timidity or boldness in children might be due to "constitutional factors," which was our way of saying that temperaments were relevant. My prior faith in the supreme power of experience had suffered its first blow.

The second source of disillusion occurred a little less than twenty years later, in the 1970s, when Richard Kearsley, Philip Zelazo, and I were summarizing our study of the effects of day care on Chinese American and Caucasian infants who either attended a day care center that we managed or were raised only at home from ages three months to twenty-nine months. To my surprise, the Chinese American infants and toddlers were quieter, more timid, and like the adult men from the Fels study who had been shy children, showed physiological signs of a more active sympathetic nervous system. These observations could be explained by acknowledging the influence of what my mother called inborn traits, which psychologists now call temperamental biases. A later chapter will document the fact that Chinese and Caucasian populations differ in many genes that have implications for temperament.

My new receptivity to the power of temperament was supported by the research of many scientists who were discovering differences among mice, rats, dogs, and monkeys from the same or related species in the tendency to approach or to avoid novel places or objects. I was also influenced by the writings of two New York psychiatrists, Alexander Thomas and Stella Chess, who surprised and irritated their psychoanalytic colleagues in the 1960s by arguing that adolescents began life with different temperaments, which they called organismic characteristics. Experience alone could not explain the personality profiles that children develop. On the basis of the parents' descriptions, Thomas and Chess suggested that infants varied on nine temperamental dimensions referring to the predictability of the infant's behaviors and moods, activity level, bias to approach or to avoid novelty, ease of adapting to new situations, energy, sensory threshold, dominant mood, distractibility, and attention span.

The combination of these events eroded my earlier prejudice and generated a desire to study temperamental biases in my laboratory. Fortunately, Cynthia Garcia-Coll, one of my graduate students who is now a professor at Brown University, was eager to pursue this idea for her thesis. She observed twenty-one-month-old children encountering unfamiliar people and objects and affirmed that some were timid and some bold. These two types preserved their tendencies into later childhood, and the timid ones showed the same sympathetic nervous system indications as the Fels adults who had been fearful three-year-olds and the Chinese American infants. Soon after, Nancy Snidman, who subsequently became a long-term colleague, made the same discovery with thirty-one-month-olds. I was now prepared, twenty-seven years after publishing *Birth to Maturity*, to take the plunge and try to prove that children like Marjorie and Lisa were born with different temperaments.

The only way to prove this idea was to observe a large group of infants, follow their development closely, and see if their infant reactions to unfamiliar intrusions could predict their later personalities in ways that made theoretical sense. Most psychologists had been reluctant to initiate such a project, for several reasons. First, most assumed, as had Thomas and Chess, that asking parents to describe their infants was as good as observing them, and it was obviously easier and less expensive. After all, they argued, mothers had more extensive knowledge of their infants than observers who could not gain information on the very large number of situations that occurred at home or could not be created in a laboratory.

However, Virginia Woolf, in a 1937 radio talk on words, captured the problem that trails reliance on language for an accurate picture of reality:

> Words . . . are the wildest, freest, most irresponsible, most unteachable of all things. . . . They are highly sensitive, easily made self-conscious. . . . They hate being useful; they hate making money . . . they hate anything that stamps them with one meaning or confines them to one attitude; for it is their nature to change.

These psychologists assumed that most parents were accurate observers of their infants' emotions and behaviors. We now know that many parents have distorted perceptions of their infants because they cannot avoid imposing an evaluation of the good or bad implications of a behavior when they describe it to a scientist. Parental descriptions emphasize the infant's irritability, regularity, ease of soothing, and expressions of pleasure or discomfort, but usually ignore the behaviors tangential to a good-bad judgment that may have a temperamental component that a camera can record, such as how long the infant plays with a toy, how often he or she smiles, or the momentary reaction to the ringing of a telephone. Equally important, parents cannot know their infant's physiology. That is why sole reliance on parental descriptions cannot be a sensitive source of information on all infant temperaments.

Finally, financial support for such projects became more difficult to obtain after 1985, because government administrators at the National Institutes of Health had decided that investigations of the genetic contributions to mental illness were more deserving of support than studies of temperamental biases that did not rest on a firm theoretical foundation. Thus, I was lucky that the MacArthur Foundation in Chicago was willing to grant me the money needed to begin the project in which Marjorie, Lisa, and more than 450 other sixteen-week-olds were enrolled from 1989 to 1991.

The mothers brought their rested and recently fed infants to my Harvard laboratory, where a woman presented them with a series of unfamiliar sights, sounds, and smells. The infants saw mobiles of brightly colored objects and stuffed animals move slowly back and forth in front of their faces, heard voices speaking sentences coming from a speaker without the presence of a person, and experienced the subtle odor of dilute alcohol on a cotton swab placed under their noses. Lisa's arms and legs remained relatively still during all of these events. Although she occasionally babbled or smiled, she rarely thrashed her arms and legs, twisted in her seat, or cried. Marjorie, by contrast, began to thrash her limbs at the third presentation of the colored mobiles and became so distressed by the fourth presentation that she lifted her back from the seat and began to cry. After Marjorie was soothed, the examiner continued. On about a third of the presentations of the mobiles, taped sentences, and the smell of alcohol, Marjorie repeated the pattern of vigorous limb movements, fretting or crying, and occasional arching of the back.

None of these episodes was frightening or frustrating, so why did these two infants react so differently? One reasonable explanation was that Marjorie and Lisa inherited a biology that affected their threshold of arousal to unfamiliar and unexpected events. If the tendencies to become highly or minimally aroused by unfamiliarity were temperamental biases that were preserved, we should see manifestations of these properties in reactions to strangers, unfamiliar rooms, and novel objects when the children were older. That is exactly what we found. Marjorie became a timid, anxious adolescent, while Lisa developed a more relaxed, spontaneous profile.

Even though the large number of human temperaments has a foundation in the child's biology, scientists do not yet know the details of that biology. Therefore, at least for now, a temperament is defined by behavior rather than by genes or brain states. Hence, we are where Darwin was when he admitted in the first edition of *Origin of Species* in 1859 that he did not know the mechanism that produced the variation in the anatomy of tortoises and finches that nature acted upon.

This book summarizes what many scientists have learned about a small number of human temperaments, especially the forms they assume during infancy, their derivatives in later childhood, their possible biological origins, the experiences that shape each set of biases into various personality types or symptoms of mental illness, and their contribution to the psychological differences between males and females and ethnic groups. I will argue, however, that no temperament is the foundation of only one personality type. Each temperament must be regarded as an initial tendency to develop one class of profiles from a large envelope of possibilities. Each bias makes it relatively easy or relatively difficult to acquire one family of behaviors, emotions, and beliefs rather than another. Thus, a personality can be likened to a gray tapestry woven from very thin black and white threads—the former representing temperaments and the latter life experiences. One sees only the gray surface and not the black and white threads. Perhaps a better metaphor for temperament is a particular block of stone in a sculptor's studio. The hardness, color, and size of the stone restrict the variety of forms the sculptor might create, while leaving the artist considerable freedom to produce a large number of aesthetic products from a particular slab of marble.

The concept of temperament, therefore, is an example of the notion of biological preparedness. Monkeys born and reared in a laboratory with no exposure to snakes will show no signs of fear the first time they see a snake. However, monkeys acquire a fear of snakes quickly if they see another animal display fear upon seeing a snake, but they do not learn to fear flowers if they see another monkey show fear behavior to a flower. It is easier to acquire a fear of snakes than a fear of flowers because the former is a biologically prepared tendency. Marjorie's temperament can be regarded as a biologically prepared tendency that makes her vulnerable to worry when a blizzard or conversation is predicted or when she has to strike up a conversation with a stranger. Lisa possesses biases that allow her to feel less threatened by the same blizzard.

Nonetheless, each child's experiences are influential. Lisa might have become a melancholic, dour adolescent if she had been born to a depressed mother and an alcoholic father who lost their tempers easily, even though these characteristics were incompatible with her initial temperament. Girls with Marjorie's temperament who grow up in poor, single-parent families in neighborhoods with high rates of crime and teenage pregnancy are at risk for becoming delinquent or pregnant, even though these traits are uncharacteristic of this bias. John Hinckley, Jr., the young man who tried to assassinate Ronald Reagan in 1987, may have possessed Marjorie's temperament, for his mother described him as an extremely anxious, timid child. It is rare that a boy with this temperament commits an aggressive act, but the frequent family moves made it difficult for him to establish lasting friendships and, in addition to other experiences that we cannot know, contributed to a personality that is uncommon in boys with this temperamental bias.

I think the Nobel laureate T. S. Eliot may have possessed Marjorie's temperament, for he was a shy, cautious, sensitive child. Most boys with this temperament do not win Nobel Prizes; however, because Eliot possessed unusual verbal abilities, in addition to the good fortune of a supportive family and attendance at good schools, he was able to exploit his temperamental preference for an introverted, solitary life to become an outstanding poet. Marjorie is verbally talented and might become a successful writer.

How Many Temperaments?

The scientists who have spent years observing infants have noted that they vary in a small number of behaviors that appear to originate in a temperament. The most obvious refer to reactions to uncomfortable states of pain, cold, and hunger. Some infants cry intensely; others do not. Among the former, some are difficult to soothe while others soothe easily. However, the intensity and duration of the cry and the ease of being soothed do not always travel together. Therefore, we can speculate that four temperamental biases are reflected in the reactions to physical distress: (1) infants who cry intensely to hunger, cold, or another source of pain and do not soothe easily, (2) infants who cry intensely but are soothed with minimal effort, (3) infants with softer cries who do not soothe easily, and finally (4) those with softer cries who are easily soothed.

The variation in infants' reactions to unfamiliar or unexpected experiences that are neither painful nor frustrating, such as new foods, textures, smells, sounds, and sights, is the basis for another quartet of temperaments. Some infants become active; others remain quiet and still. Some cry; others are quiet. These reactions to novel events generate four additional temperaments: (1) infants who display vigorous movements and cry frequently, (2) those who display vigorous movements but rarely cry, (3) those who remain still but cry, and finally (4) those who remain still and rarely cry. Marjorie belongs to the first category, which I call high-reactive, whereas Lisa belongs to the fourth category, called low-reactive.

Infants also vary in their reaction to frustrations—for example, losing the nipple they were sucking, dropping or failing to retrieve a toy, or being restrained by a blanket or an adult's hands. The combinations of movements and crying that occur to unfamiliarity also occur in frustration, yielding an additional set of four temperaments. Finally, infants vary in the frequency of spontaneous babbling, smiling, or limb movements when they are simply lying in a crib with no intrusions. This variation adds three more temperaments.

These fifteen biases are defined by infants' behavior, not by their private feelings, because scientists cannot measure the latter at the present time. However, it is likely that infants also vary in the intensity of pleasure they experience to events such as sweet tastes and gentle caresses, and in the intensity of the unpleasant state provoked by events that include bitter tastes and rough handling. Young infants display a distinctive facial response to bitter or sour tastes. They often curl their upper lip, wrinkle their nose, and stick out their tongue. When this facial pattern occurs to the foul taste of rotten food or the smell of feces, we assume the individuals are experiencing the unpleasant emotion of disgust. However, only a minority of school-age children displayed these facial responses to the smell of feces. Indeed, a majority of girls smiled to the odor of feces if they were with an unfamiliar examiner in a laboratory setting, as if to communicate to the adult that they recognized the inappropriateness of the smell in this context. Thus these facial reactions are not automatic reflexes in older individuals.

A caretaker's temporary absence can evoke fretting, which is regarded as a sign of fear; a turning down of the mouth in the form of a frown, which is regarded as a sign of sadness; or a loud cry and a wide-open mouth, which is treated as a sign of anger. These four behavioral profiles are associated with four brain patterns that probably create different unpleasant feelings in the infant. The developing brain-mind builds on these early brain-mind states to create the emotions we call disgust, fear, sadness, and anger in older children. If infants varied in the excitability of each of the four circuits, due to genes or prenatal events, they might be expected to vary in their later susceptibility to these emotions.

A similar argument can be made for the pleasant states induced by sweet tastes, playing "peekaboo" with a parent, the successful completion of a block tower, and the receipt of physical affection. The special quality of "pleasure" evoked by each of these different events originates in distinctive brain circuits and neurochemistries. Therefore, these experiences in infancy and early childhood could be the foundation of the emotions that we call sensory delight, excitement, pride, and joy in older individuals. As with the four unpleasant feeling states, infants might vary in the excitability of each of these circuits and, therefore, in their vulnerability to the relevant emotions when they are older.

Thus, future investigators may add these eight biases to the fifteen that are more easily detected by observing a large number of infants and measuring their brain states. However, twenty-three is a small number in light of the much larger number of possible temperaments that could have a biological foundation. I suspect scientists will discover that most, but not all, biases have their origin in inherited patterns of chemical molecules and associated receptors that affect brain activity.

Molecules and Genes

The brain is influenced by more than 150 molecules, many of which facilitate or inhibit the transfer of information over the narrow synaptic space between neurons. Some of the frequently studied molecules are called dopamine, norepinephrine, serotonin, acetylcholine, oxytocin, vasopressin, and opioids. Each molecule has a special affinity for and power to activate particular protein receptors lying on the surface of neurons. A second class of molecules reduces the duration of excitatory activity by destroying the excitatory molecule or returning it to its source. The relation between a molecule and its receptors can be likened to the relation between the ridges of a key and the internal shape of the lock into which it fits. When these molecules attach to their assigned receptors, a cascade of reactions occurs, resulting in activation or inhibition of neurons, and as a result a particular brain state is established that could be the foundation of a temperament.

The concentration of each molecule and the number and location of the receptors are under the control of specific genes. Each gene is a string of DNA comprising repetitions of pairs of four molecules (called bases, with the names adenine, guanine, cytosine, and thymine). Each base is attached to a sugar and a phosphate molecule, and this more complex structure is called a nucleotide. Some genes, called structural genes, are the origin of the amino acids that are used to synthesize the proteins that are the building blocks of our bodies. Others, called promoters and enhancers, regulate the structural genes; still other strings (introns) are located within the structural gene but are deleted when these strings are transferred from the nucleus of the cell to structures in the cell's larger area (called cytoplasm) that make proteins. A typical gene is composed of about 100,000 nucleotides.

Each of the three types of strings can have more than one base in exactly the same place in the string. When more than one base is in the same location, biologists say that this location represents an "allele" of the gene. Although an allele of an original gene can be established in many ways, four changes are particularly common. If, for illustration, one sequence of bases was A-B-C-D, an allele could be the result of: (1) a reversal of the sequence, as in D-C-B-A, (2) a deletion of a base, as in A-C-D, (3) the insertion of a base, as in A-C-D-B-C, or (4) the repetition of a base, as in A-B-C-D-D-D-D. I make this idea concrete with a real example. Most living forms possess a protein important in respiration that has remained relatively stable over time. The gene that is the foundation of the amino acids that are combined to construct this protein consists of a string of 312 bases. Humans and monkeys differ in only 1 of the 312, humans and dogs differ in 13, and humans and moths differ in 36 of the bases.

Words, which are strings of letters, provide a helpful analogy. If "love" was the original word then "evol," "lve," "loeve," and "loveeee" would be "alleles" of the original word. Moreover, just as genes can change over the course of a lifetime, words can change their meaning and spelling over the course of centuries. The term "economics," which refers to the science dealing with the production and consumption of goods, is derived from the Latin word *oeconomica*, which originally meant "family life." The analogy extends to the significance of location. The products of a gene depend on where it is located in the body; the meaning of a word, too, depends on the social context in which it is spoken. The word "bad" in the phrase "it was bad" could refer to an unhappy experience, a poor performance, or a severe storm. Finally, most single changes in any one of the four bases have no effect on the functioning of the organism. They are analogous to deleting certain phonemes of a word when speaking; no one would have a problem understanding a person who said, "I am goin' home" rather than "I am going home."

If we are conservative and assume, first, that only 200 of the 30,000 structural genes (less than 2 percent of the genome) are the foundation of the molecules and receptors that contribute to human temperaments (actually 50 percent of human genes affect brain activity) and, second, that each gene has only four alleles (many genes have more than four), there could potentially be two thousand biologically distinct temperaments. This number is much larger than the twenty-three temperaments described earlier. These facts pose a paradox: Why have psychologists observed such a small number of temperamental biases when, potentially, there could be close to two thousand?

First, it is possible that many of the two thousand genetic patterns have no implications for a temperament, even though they contribute to a brain state. Second, there are probably many subtypes within each of the biases. Perhaps some infants scream at the pain of a diaper pin piercing their skin but do not cry intensely when they are hungry. Some infants might cry when an unfamiliar person approaches but remain calm when fed an unfamiliar food. Some infants may smile when they see their mothers but not when they encounter the game of peekaboo. Third, I noted that some biases affect sensations that are too subtle to observe. For example, some individuals have a larger than expected number of taste buds for sweet or bitter substances. As a result, they experience a more intense sensation from tasting ice cream or turnips. Fourth, in some cases the psychological profile that develops depends on whether the child inherited the gene from the mother or the father. Finally, a particular psychological trait could be the product of a special temperamental bias combined with experience or a history of life experiences without a special bias. Scientists who place individuals in a scanner that measures patterns of blood flow to various brain locations often discover that individuals who performed equally well on a task differ in blood flow patterns while working on the task. Although each of these plausible explanations reduces the imbalance between the large number of possible biological states and the smaller number of known temperaments, the imbalance remains. I suspect that future research will reveal many, many more temperaments than the twenty-three candidates I nominated. However, even when scientists discover the genes that predispose a child to a particular temperament, it will still be impossible to predict the personality that the adult will possess because there are too many ways to create the same adult pattern of acts, beliefs, moods, and acute emotions. A letter sent from London can take many different routes before arriving at its destination in San Francisco. Thus, we need to know more than a person's genes and temperaments to predict the adult personality. Many scientists are trying to discover these facts.

At the present time, however, no scientist has discovered any gene, or set of genes, that is always associated with a particular temperament, mood, or symptom of mental illness independent of the person's gender, life experiences, and ethnicity. For example, possession of an allele affecting serotonin activity in the brain can lead to social anxiety in a middle-class female raised by affectionate parents, but it can lead to criminality in a male who was reared in poverty by neglecting parents. One team of scientists trying to predict the occurrence of a bout of depression from the presence of an allele controlling serotonin activity had to know the person's gender, ethnicity (black or white), and whether he or she had been experiencing serious life stress in order to predict who became depressed. Knowing that the person had the allele was insufficient.

The same is true for monkeys observed under highly controlled conditions. Infant monkeys with different alleles of a gene responsible for a molecule affecting brain states were raised under different conditions. When the scientists measured behavioral signs of fear to an unfamiliar human approaching the animal's living area, they found no consistent effect of any of the alleles on behavior. But the monkeys that were raised with only their mothers, and no other animals, were the most fearful, independent of the allele they inherited. That is, the monkey's life history had more influence than its genes on the level of fear of the unfamiliar human. The same conclusion holds for adults who experience a harsh childhood. The harsh conditions are usually more influential than any particular allele, although the combination of a harsh home environment and a relevant allele is sometimes a better predictor of depression or anxiety than either the gene or the life conditions considered alone. Predicting which adults would develop serious anxiety following a severe hurricane in Florida was possible only if the scientists took into account the person's gender (female), whether he or she lacked social support, and whether he or she possessed a particular gene. Possession of only one of these features did not predict the level of anxiety. That is why Barry Barnes and John Dupré, who wrote *Genomes and What to Make of Them*, reminded us that DNA is not the master molecule but a molecule that scientists have mastered. It is important to appreciate that only sixty years ago most scientists would have rejected the suggestion that brain activity was influenced in a major way by molecules originating in particular genes. Thus we are in an early stage of understanding the relations among genes, brain chemistry, and psychological phenomena; it is analogous to our understanding of the universe when Galileo and Kepler declared that the earth revolved around the sun.

Other Origins of Temperament

Although inherited variation in brain chemistry may be the most frequent basis for a temperament, it is not the only source. Identical twins do not have identical fingerprints, and the first kitten that was cloned from one of its mother's cells (and therefore was genetically identical to the mother) had a coat color and personality that differed from the comparable features in the mother.

The month when a child is conceived might contribute in a small way to a select number of temperaments because the pregnant woman's physiology is influenced by changes in the hours of daylight that occur during the spring and fall. When daylight is decreasing faster than usual, from late August to late October in the Northern Hemisphere, humans secrete larger amounts of a molecule called melatonin, and women differ in the amount of melatonin they secrete as dusk approaches each day. Fetuses conceived during the interval from late February through late May, when the hours of daylight are increasing, are exposed to smaller amounts of maternal melatonin than those conceived from late August through late October. Melatonin has profound influences on the brain and body of the mother and in turn on the developing embryo, including the activation or silencing of genes, increased antioxidant activity, and the synthesis of molecules that influence the still-undeveloped brain. These facts make it reasonable to speculate that embryos possessing genes that render them especially vulnerable to higher or lower concentrations of melatonin will be affected by their month of conception.

Children conceived during the spring months in the Northern Hemisphere are at a higher risk for becoming schizophrenic. Those conceived during the fall months are at a slightly higher risk for extreme shyness during childhood, depression or suicidal thinking during adulthood, and disorders of the immune system, including multiple sclerosis. Adults who become unusually apathetic during the winter months, when the hours of daylight are reduced, have a much smaller rise in the stress hormone cortisol during the first hour after awakening compared with most adults, whose large rise in cortisol contributes to a heightened alertness and arousal. Although the magnitude of risk for any of these undesirable outcomes is small in an absolute sense, it is nonetheless real. The astrologers who ascribed personality traits to individuals on the basis of the arrangement of stars and planets during the month they were born had a good idea but a wildly incorrect explanation.

Unusual conditions present during pregnancy can also contribute to temperament. Maternal infections, extreme stress, serious abuse of alcohol or drugs during pregnancy, or the number of prior pregnancies that delivered boys can create conditions in the womb or at birth that lead to chemical, anatomical, or immune disturbances that, in turn, create psychological biases in infants. For example, Canadian mothers who had been exposed to a severe ice storm in 1998 when their fetuses were in the second trimester were more likely to bear babies who had different fingerprint patterns on corresponding fingers, which is a sign of disturbed development often found in adults with schizophrenia. Infants born to mothers who abused alcohol during pregnancy often have disturbed brain functions and behavior. Almost 15 percent of American women of childbearing age (more than 7 million women) admitted to engaging in binge drinking during 2001. The true number is probably larger. One consequence of heavy alcohol consumption during pregnancy is subtle differences between the right and left sides of the baby's face. These asymmetries include the width of the eye, the distance between the pupil of the eye and the top of the nose, and the distance between the cheekbone and the corner of the mouth. American and European adults with only slightly different values on these measures on the left and right sides of the face are judged less attractive, have their first sexual experience later, and have fewer sexual partners during the adult years. The most celebrated female film stars and models for cosmetics have unusually symmetrical faces.

Unborn infants whose mothers have been exposed to the flu during their pregnancy are at a slightly higher risk for developing schizophrenia later in life because the mother's immune system responds to the infection by producing molecules (called cytokines) that affect the developing fetus. The elegant research of Paul Patterson of the California Institute of Technology has revealed that mice born to mothers who had been infected with the flu virus while pregnant were more reluctant than the average mouse to explore an unfamiliar place, suggesting that these animals had an exaggerated reaction to novel locations. In addition, human infants who are exposed to extreme trauma or serious infection during the first year of life can develop particular temperaments because their immature brains are vulnerable to select stressors.

Severely premature infants (less than four or five pounds at birth) can develop distinct emotional or behavioral profiles during the first few years of life.

One of the most intriguing processes operating before and during birth involves the number of older brothers that preceded the birth of a particular boy. The Y chromosome, unique to males, contains proteins that the mother's body treats as foreign (called antigens), and the pregnant woman produces antibodies against these proteins. When the blood of the newborn and the mother mix at the time of birth, the mother's antibodies against the male proteins are introduced into the bloodstream of the newborn infant. The firstborn male escapes this potentially harmful immune reaction, but every successive male infant is at increasing risk for an immune reaction that can alter his brain. A similar mechanism is operative when the fetus and the mother have different blood types. One of the possible consequences of the mother's antibodies against these proteins has some preliminary support. Later-born males who have several older brothers have a slightly higher probability of developing a gay lifestyle, but only if they are also right-handed. It is not known why left-handed males with older brothers are not affected in the same way by this immune response.

Finally, Peter Pharoah, of the University of Liverpool, estimates that in 3 to 5 percent of all single births the parents were unaware of the fact that a twin sibling had died early in the pregnancy. The surviving child, whose anatomy or physiology could have been affected by the embryo that did not survive, is at a slightly higher risk for abnormal traits, some of which might be temperamental biases.

It is useful to distinguish among the different reasons for an observed temperamental bias, and I will try in the rest of the book to specify the origin of the bias. For example, although both the humans who migrated to Tibet 25,000 years ago and those who settled in the Andes mountains about 10,000 years later had physiologies that were adapted to high altitudes, each group developed different mechanisms to accomplish the same aim. Although I suspect that neurochemical profiles will turn out to be the most frequent reasons for the biases found in a majority of children, I acknowledge that other mechanisms might create similar temperamental profiles.

Societies pass through historical cycles in which one idea temporarily dominates its complement until the former overreaches its legitimate power and is replaced with a sister perspective. The nineteenth century's romance with emotion replaced the hyper-rationality of the previous century. The unchallenged celebration of a laissez-faire economy, promoted by Adam Smith in 1776, had to be checked a century later by governmental regulations that restricted the exploitation of the many by the few. Many psychologists and psychiatrists are currently emphasizing the power of biology as a balance to the unrealistically ambitious claims made by the scholars who were certain that experience was the sovereign sculptor of human variation. It will take a while before scientists acknowledge once again the complementary contributions of biology and experience. The cycles of changing beliefs in a society resemble a child who is continually off balance as he or she walks on the top of a picket fence.

The scientific advances made since my years as a graduate student have eroded my earlier resistance to the significant effects of biology on development. Very few social scientists continue to insist that experience alone could have generated the distinctive personalities possessed by Marjorie and Lisa. The concept of a temperamental bias is necessary to help explain why siblings from the same family or adolescents who grew up in very similar homes have different personalities. But the advances of the last fifty years have also revealed the extraordinary complexity of these biological biases and the need to combine biology with experience in order to explain a person's characteristic moods, reactions to challenge, and daily habits. We have rejected the earlier dogma that assigned total power to nurture, but we are unsure of which path to take as we attempt to illuminate the many remaining mysteries.

2

Reacting to
the Unexpected

The sudden siren of a fire engine, flickering of a lamp, or cramp from a muscle are only a few examples of the many events that automatically shift the focus of attention because they are unexpected. If the event is familiar and free of threat, which is true of most unexpected experiences, the mind quickly returns to its prior concerns. However, when an unexpected event is also unfamiliar, it may be treated as a possible sign of danger requiring a vigilant posture, flight, or preparation for a defensive maneuver. Some temperaments affect the quality, intensity, and duration of the reactions to unexpected or unfamiliar events.

Two brain structures—the amygdala and the prefrontal cortex— orchestrate the person's response to the unexpected (figure 1). The adage "Big things come in small packages" is especially appropriate for the amygdala. This relatively small structure in the middle of the brain, close to the temporal cortex, contains at least five specialized neuronal clusters. But the most important fact is that some of these neurons respond to any unexpected or unfamiliar event, whether dangerous or benign, and alert other neurons in the amygdala, as well as other brain sites, to react appropriately. Not surprisingly, some parts of the amygdala receive sensory information from the outside world as well as from the body. The individual, human or animal, continually uses this information to create an expectation of what might happen in the next moment. If the event of the next moment violates that expectation, neurons in the amygdala and nearby cortex are activated within one-fifth of a second, which is a full one-fifth of a second before the brain detects the meaning of the event. The trigger for the amygdala under these circumstances is not a specific event but the comparison between some salient features of the event and the expectation created by the immediate past. Other neurons in the amygdala activate sites in the prefrontal cortex that judge the possibility of a threat, and still other sites initiate behavioral and physiological reactions designed to protect the individual from possible danger. Should the prefrontal cortex evaluate the event as safe, it will send signals back to the amygdala to block the preparations for fight or flight—as, for example, an American president decides to abort a nuclear weapon being readied for firing in a military installation thousands of miles away. The reciprocal relation between the prefrontal cortex and the amygdala is one example of the exquisite balance between excitation and inhibition that is found in many places in the brain.

Humans, as well as animals, differ in the excitability of their amygdala and, therefore, in their reactions to unexpected or unfamiliar events. About one of seven house cats is extremely timid. They fail to explore unfamiliar places, retreat from a stranger, and usually do not attack rats. This timidity emerges at about two months of age (comparable to about fourteen months in a human

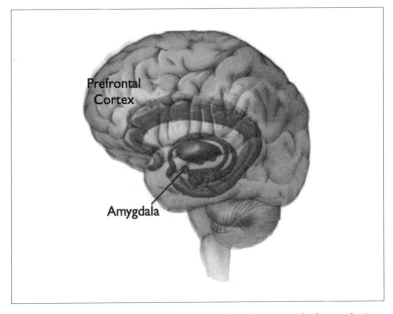

Figure 1. The location of the amygdala and prefrontal cortex in the human brain.

infant), and the amygdalae of the timid kittens become unusually excited when they hear sounds that resemble the threat howl of an adult cat. Because measuring variation in amygdalar excitability directly requires placing infants in a magnetic scanner, an expensive and stressful procedure that many parents of healthy infants might refuse, most psychologists have to settle for measuring indirect signs of this property in the child's behavior.

Most species have a preferred behavioral reaction to unexpected events. A squirrel scampering on a lawn stops in its tracks if it hears a sound; a dog barks at the sight of an unfamiliar person. We filmed the behaviors of more than 450 infants, including Marjorie and Lisa, as they responded to unexpected stimuli. These four-month-olds, whom my colleagues and I have been studying for about twenty years, were born healthy to married, financially secure white mothers who did not smoke, take illicit drugs, or drink alcohol to excess during their pregnancies. The restriction to white infants was necessary because Africans, Hispanics, and Asians inherit a brain chemistry that is slightly different from the brain chemistry of Caucasians. In chapter 5, I'll explain in more detail how interesting these slight differences turn out to be.

The infants were presented with colorful moving mobiles, taped human voices, and a cotton swab dipped in diluted alcohol and applied to the nostrils. None of these experiences was harmful or painful, only unexpected and unfamiliar. We assumed that the four-month-old human infants whose amygdala was especially sensitive to unexpected or unfamiliar events would thrash their arms and legs and cry, not because they were afraid but because their amygdala overreacted to a stimulus they either did not expect or did not know.

Four Kinds of Infants

About 20 percent of the infants—one in five—reacted distinctively to the unexpected events. These infants, called *high-reactive*, thrashed their arms and legs and cried on about a third of the presentations and, on several occasions, arched their back by lifting it from the cushioned seat on which they rested. The arching of the back is an important clue because the central nucleus of the amygdala communicates with a neuronal cluster in the brain stem that mediates this infrequent but distinctive response. This same cluster is activated when adults anticipate physical harm. Therefore, infants who arch their backs to unexpected events probably have a more excitable amygdala.

The 40 percent who displayed the opposite profile, called *low-reactive*, usually remained still, rarely cried or arched their backs, and often babbled or smiled. The remaining infants belonged to one of two other groups. About one in four did not move much but cried a lot (called *distressed*); one in ten moved their arms and legs and often smiled and babbled, but rarely cried or arched their backs (called *aroused*). The remaining 5 percent were difficult to classify. I am relatively confident about these proportions because Nathan Fox of the University of Maryland, who repeated the same procedures with an equally large group of Maryland infants, found the same four types in roughly similar proportions.

Later Development of High- and Low-reactives

The critical question is whether high- and low-reactive infants display distinctive behavioral, emotional, and biological profiles in later childhood. If they do, we can be relatively confident that the behaviors shown at sixteen weeks were sensitive signs of two temperamental biases. Fortunately, this question has an affirmative answer.

The infants returned to our laboratory when they were about one and two years old to encounter a variety of unfamiliar adults, rooms, objects, and procedures on an unpredictable schedule with their mothers always nearby. Young children show signs of fear to three kinds of experiences. One is an intrusion into their personal space—for example, the placement of electrodes on their body or a blood pressure cuff on their arm. Unfamiliar objects or movements also generate fear, and we presented the children with robots, toy animals, puppets, flashing lights, and the unexpected appearance of a toy clown striking a drum. Finally, young children become apprehensive when they encounter unfamiliar people, especially those who assume unfamiliar facial expressions or wear novel costumes. By exploiting all three types of unfamiliarity, we could be more certain that the children who showed a fear reaction to two or all three types had a temperament that disposed them to cry or to retreat from unfamiliar experiences that they had not anticipated.

The episodes that produced an immediate cry of fear in most children were the application of electrodes or a blood pressure cuff, a rotating wheel that generated an unusual noise, the placement of a drop of liquid on the child's tongue, and the stern voice and frown of a female examiner showing the child a rotating toy. Other procedures provoked an avoidant reaction but not always crying. These included occasions when the child refused to touch an unfamiliar toy or approach a stranger or a woman dressed in a clown costume and mask who invited the child in a friendly voice to join her in play.

About one-third of the one- and two-year-olds displayed no fear or only one fear to the seventeen unfamiliar episodes; another third showed two or three fears; and a final third displayed four or more fears. We classified children as minimally fearful if they displayed no more than one fear and as highly fearful if they displayed four or more fears. As we expected, a majority of the one- and two-year-olds who had been high-reactive infants were highly fearful, whereas a majority of those who had been low-reactive were minimally fearful. The other two groups displayed intermediate levels of fear. We learned from a later study of twins living in Colorado that these differences in timid behavior in the second year are partially influenced by genes. In 1946, Donald Hebb wrote an important paper on fear in which he noted that about one-third of the chimpanzees housed in a Florida field station became very fearful to the presentation of unfamiliar objects, such as the replica of a head of a chimpanzee, a doll, and a skull.

Marjorie was one of the high-reactive children who was highly fearful at fourteen months. She cried when placed on a rug in an unfamiliar room during a warm-up period (less than 5 percent of infants cried during this initial episode); when the examiner tried to put electrodes on her chest or place a blood pressure cuff around her arm; and when the examiner spoke in a stern voice with a frown on her face. She refused to put her hand into a cup of black liquid, would not accept the liquid on her tongue, and ran to her mother when a stranger entered the playroom.

At twenty-one months of age Marjorie refused to play with some unfamiliar toys and when the examiner modeled a block construction and invited her to imitate, she said, "I can't do it." She retreated to her mother when an unfamiliar woman entered the room and invited Marjorie to play and remained close to the parent until the stranger left. When a person in a clown costume entered the room unexpectedly, Marjorie raced to her mother, sobbing repeatedly, "No, no, no."

By contrast, Lisa was one of the small proportion of low-reactive infants who displayed no fears at either age. She squealed with laughter to many episodes, greeted the stranger, threw a toy at the clown, and approached the moving toy robot immediately. Her mother commented that her behaviors in the laboratory resembled her demeanor at home.

When the children were 4½ years old they participated in a play session with two other unfamiliar children of the same sex and age while the three parents sat on a couch in the same room. Twice as many low-reactives as high-reactives were sociable and talkative, whereas about 50 percent of high-reactives were shy, quiet, and spent long periods of time standing close to their mothers.

Sara Rimm-Kaufman, who is now at the University of Virginia, observed some of these children four times during their kinder-garten year between the first week of September, when school began, and in late January. More high- than low-reactives were quiet, refused to volunteer when the teacher invited a response, rarely broke the teacher's rules against whispering or yelling, and were reluctant to approach Sara, who stood quietly in the back of the room. The low-reactives often volunteered comments, yelled, and more than half of them approached Sara at least once during her visits.

When the children were seven years old, we asked the mothers and teachers about the occurrence of signs of fear, shyness, or timidity. Children were classified as anxious if they met two criteria: The parents had to report four or more signs of anxiety from a list that included requiring a night light when sleeping, refusing to stay overnight at a friend's house, displaying fear of large animals or storms, or asking a parent whether they or the parent might die. In addition, the teacher had to rank the child as among the most timid in the classroom. Although only 20 percent of the original group had been high-reactive, 45 percent with this temperament as babies were classified as anxious at age seven. Many of these children had screamed in fear five years earlier when the clown unexpectedly entered the playroom. Forty percent of the original study group had been low-reactive but at age seven less than 15 percent of this group possessed signs of anxiety. About one of five high-reactives were consistently timid, shy, and quiet during the evaluations at one, two, four, and seven years of age, but not one low-reactive maintained a subdued, timid profile during all four assessments.

Nathan Fox and Kenneth Rubin of the University of Maryland, whose observations of comparable groups of children yielded similar results, discovered that very shy, reticent two-year-olds who have intrusive or overprotective mothers are most likely to remain timid and anxious. Those with less-demanding parents, as well as those who attended a well-run day care center, were less fearful. Among children who were still timid when it was time to begin school, the shy, timid boys were at greater risk for being teased and rejected by peers than were the shy girls, because boys are cruel to those boys who violate the sex-role stereotype demanding control of fear. Girls are gentler with friends who appear anxious and, as a result, shy girls have an easier time overcoming their public timidity.

We saw these children again in 2000 and 2001, when they were eleven years old. As anticipated, a larger proportion of high-reactives than low-reactives were quiet and serious while conversing with the examiner, whereas many low-reactives were garrulous, had a relaxed posture, and smiled and laughed frequently. A different, but equally unfamiliar, woman interviewed them in their homes when they were fifteen years old. The adolescents who had been high-reactive fidgeted with their hair and face, rarely smiled, and failed to elaborate their answers to the interviewer's questions. Spontaneous smiling was a sensitive sign of their infant temperament. High-reactives were less likely to smile during every assessment, from four months to fifteen years, whereas a majority of low-reactives punctuated their conversations with the examiner with frequent smiles and laughter at every age.

The content of adolescent worries revealed an important difference between the two temperamental groups. Although all of these middle-class adolescents said they occasionally worried about examinations, grades, and their performance on the athletic field or in the concert hall, two-thirds of the high-reactives, but only 20 percent of the low-reactives, reported less realistic worries, over events, such as talking with a stranger, being in a crowd, visiting an unfamiliar city, riding on a subway, or thinking about their future. The quality of anxiety provoked by concern over a final examination or performance on a soccer field differs from the quality that accompanies worrying over a visit to Washington, D.C., talking with a stranger, or brooding about the uncertainty implicit in the future. Here are some typical statements of high-reactives: "In a crowd I feel isolated and left out;" "I don't know what to pay attention to because it is all so ambiguous;" "I worry about the future, not knowing what will happen next;" "I wanted to be a doctor but decided against it because I felt it would be too much of a strain;" "I like being alone, and I don't have to worry about fitting in with others when I am with my horse;" "I get nervous before every vacation because I don't know what will happen." One high-reactive girl told the interviewer she did not like spring because the weather was unpredictable.

These statements imply that their earlier vulnerability to uncertainty following encounters with unfamiliar events had expanded to include uncertainty about which action to choose when alternatives were possible. The former situation evokes event uncertainty; the latter creates response uncertainty. Adults who experience the latter state frequently report that they feel frustrated and stressed when they do not have all the information they need to make a decision, and they dislike being unable to predict the future. Youth who are unusually anxious about the future, the ethical values they should honor, or meeting people they do not know are likely to retain these worries for years. High-reactive youth feel more comfortable when the rules are clear and the differences between right and wrong are free of ambiguity. Unfortunately, this cohort of American adolescents lives at a time when there is a great deal of ambiguity about required sexual behaviors, degree of loyalty to friends, and life goals. The uncertainty created by this ethical confusion is more intense in high- than in low-reactives, for the former find it harder to live in a community where "anything goes." It is not surprising, therefore, that more high- than low-reactives are deeply religious, despite no difference between the two groups in the religiosity of their parents. Many high-reactives told the interviewer that their religious commitment eased their tension by providing clear guides for action and a friendly group of peers who shared their moral beliefs. Many American adolescents and adults without any temperamental bias for anxiety are aware of the ambiguity surrounding the ethical standards that must be honored, and the proportion affiliated with a church, especially among those without a professional degree, has risen over the past fifty years.

At the end of the three-hour interview in the home, the woman gave each fifteen-year-old a set of twenty cards, each describing a personality trait; for example, "I often wonder what my friends think of me," "I worry about getting a bad grade," "Most of the time I'm happy," "I'm shy with adults I don't know." Each youth ranked the twenty statements in accord with how well the description characterized his or her personality. Five other descriptions reflected a dour, melancholic mood: "I am pretty serious," "I think too much before deciding what to do," "I wish I were more relaxed," and denial of the statement "I'm easygoing." The high-reactives were far more likely than low-reactives to endorse the serious, dour traits as characteristic of themselves. By contrast, most low-reactives described themselves as happy, easygoing, and relaxed. Our observations of these youth affirm their self-descriptions and support our belief in a temperamental contribution to a lighthearted mood or a dour one. The serious youth are vulnerable to bodily sensations, such as a fast-beating heart, a growling stomach, or difficulty breathing. The sudden intrusion of these feelings, along with an inability to understand them, provokes anxiety, and adults with this trait are regarded as having high anxiety sensitivity. The persistence of a dour or lighthearted mood reminds me of a cartoon in the *New Yorker* magazine illustrating two men talking on the lawn of a large mansion with a luxury car, swimming pool, and horse in the background. The caption had one man saying, "I could cry when I think of the years I wasted accumulating money, only to learn that my cheerful disposition is genetic."

The Biological Signs

We measured four biological reactions at eleven and fifteen years of age that are indirect signs of the excitability of the amygdala. One was the activity of neurons in a small site in the brain called the inferior colliculus, an early component of a circuit that transmits sound from the outer ear to the auditory cortex. Neurons in varied brain locations have preferred rates of firing, analogous to the usual vibration frequencies of the strings of a harp, piano, or guitar. This firing rate is increased when the neuron is stimulated, either by an external event or by input from another brain structure. We recorded the level of activation of the inferior colliculus because the amgydala sends impulses to this site. A person with a more excitable amygdala should have a more excitable inferior colliculus and, therefore, a larger response to sound as indexed by the amplitude of the wave detected in the electroencephalogram (figure 2). We recorded the magnitude of activity in this structure while the adolescent was sitting quietly and listening to click sounds through headphones. Forty percent of the high-reactives, but not one low-reactive, displayed evidence of a highly excitable colliculus at both eleven and fifteen years of age, suggesting that the high-reactives had a more aroused amygdala.

Another way to evaluate the excitability of the amygdala is to measure the brain's reaction to unfamiliar pictures that could not be anticipated, such as a chair with one leg or the body of an animal with the head of an infant. Unexpected events, especially if they are unfamiliar, activate the basolateral area of the

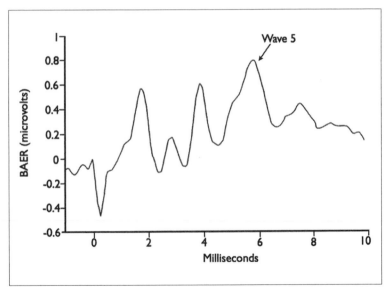

Figure 2. The waveform of the brain stem auditory evoked response. The arrow points to the waveform from the inferior colliculus.

amygdala, which, in turn, excites neurons in the temporal and frontal lobes. The coherent firing of large numbers of neurons in the latter two structures produces a distinct brain wave, about four-tenths of a second after the onset of the event, whose magnitude is related to the excitability of the amygdala (figure 3). As anticipated, all the adolescents had a distinctive brain wave to the unfamiliar pictures (called Nc in the figure). But the high-reactives had a much larger wave than the low-reactives, implying that their amygdala was more responsive to pictures that were both unexpected and discrepant from their prior experience.

We also took advantage of the fact that neuronal clusters have preferred firing rates. When a person is relaxed, neither buried

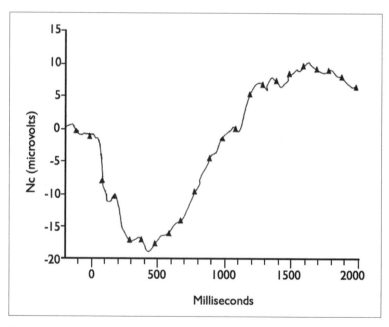

Figure 3. A typical event-related potential waveform to an unexpected or unfamiliar event. Note that the largest magnitudes occur between 300 and 600 milliseconds.

in thought nor solving a problem, large numbers of neurons in many parts of the brain fire together at a rate approximating ten times a second—imagine a chorus line of millions of dancers all moving their legs together at the same frequency. The neuron's firing rate at a particular site increases when it receives input from another structure.

Activity in the body, from heart, gut, and muscles, ascends through a connected set of structures to many sites in the brain, including the amygdala. The amount of activity transmitted from body to brain is usually greater on the right side than on the left side; therefore, the amygdala in the right hemisphere should be more excited than the amygdala on the left in individuals with a great deal of activity in heart, blood vessels, muscle groups, and gut. The amygdalar neurons in each hemisphere relay their activity to select sites in the frontal lobe of the same hemisphere. About two-thirds of adolescents and adults have greater activation in the left compared with the right side of the frontal lobe. These individuals often report that they are happy and relaxed. The smaller group, which shows more activity in the frontal lobe of the right hemisphere, is more likely to report frequent episodes of unhappiness, tension, and anxiety.

More high- than low-reactives showed greater activation of the right compared with the left frontal lobe at both eleven and fifteen years; more low-reactives showed the opposite pattern. Nathan Fox has reported that the high-reactives in his sample who were very shy at fourteen, twenty-four, and twenty-eight months were also likely to show greater activation of the right frontal lobe.

A final sign of a reactive amygdala was revealed in the child's heart rate patterns. The central area of the amygdala sends information to sites in the sympathetic nervous system that control heart rate and its variability. High-reactives were more likely than low-reactives to show a heart rate pattern suggestive of a more active sympathetic nervous system. This pattern resembled the one we saw in 1962 in the Fels adults who had been timid children. High-reactives also had warmer fingertips than low-reactives because the temperature of the fingertips is higher in individuals with higher heart rates. The heightened sympathetic activity of the high-reactives was also present at one year. These children displayed a very large increase in heart rate when the examiner put a drop of lemon juice on their tongue. Thus, all four indirect signs of amygdalar excitability at eleven and fifteen years differentiated the adolescents who had been high- or low-reactive at sixteen weeks of age.

A lack of confidence about the correct behavior to display, a state called response uncertainty, also activates the amygdala. Anxious adolescents showed greater amygdalar activity to faces with fearful expressions than normal youth did when they had to judge how afraid they were of the faces, because they did not know how to answer that request. When the adolescents were simply looking at the fearful faces and did not have to decide on their emotion, there was no difference in amygdalar activity between anxious and non-anxious groups. Similarly, anxious adults showed equivalent levels of amygdalar excitability during the few seconds before an unpleasant scene (a mutilated body) or a neutral picture (a plate) appeared on a screen, because they (the anxious adults) were not sure what they would see. This is not an original insight. Benjamin Franklin suggested that "uneasiness" was a significant human emotion because unexpected events are more often unwanted than desired. So when we do not know what might happen in the next few moments or hours, we are more likely to be apprehensive than when we are eagerly antici-pating a pleasant surprise.

The amygdala is also activated when a person recognizes that he or she has made a mistake on a task. Although all children make errors in school, at home, and on the playground, high-reac-tive children have a much larger amygdalar response, because the brain's reaction to the error is added to their usually high level of excitability. As a result, they are likely to experience a rise in heart rate and muscle tension and interpret these feelings as meaning they are anxious. Because the state of the amygdala is influenced by a large number of molecules, and there are many different ways to produce an excitable amygdala, it is impossible, at least at present, to name the genes or molecules that might contribute to this brain state in the adolescents or adults who had been high-reactive infants.

In addition, more high- than low-reactives had an allergy to pollen, and two-thirds of the high-reactives had at least one parent who had hay fever. A susceptibility to allergies can result from greater activity in the sympathetic nervous system, which suppresses the integrity of the immune system. It is relevant, therefore, that children with a parent who suffered either from an anxiety disorder characterized by unexpected panic attacks or from serious depression were more likely than the average child to have an allergy.

The slightly higher prevalence of blue eyes among high-reac-tives in this all-Caucasian group was a second intriguing fact. This observation matched one reported by Allison Rosenberg, who asked the teachers of 133 classrooms (from kindergarten to third grade) to nominate, from all the Caucasian pupils in their classes, the single child who was the shyest and the one who was most sociable. More extremely shy children had blue eyes; more extremely sociable children had brown eyes. A small group of ten very shy girls, who were members of a larger group of 148 Caucasians, had a high heart rate, a mother who suffered from panic disorder, and light blue eyes. We shall see in chapter 5 that Caucasian adults living in northern latitudes—for example, Sweden and Norway—are more likely to have blue eyes and a more reactive sympathetic nervous system than those living in the more southern latitudes of Italy and Greece.

A final pair of observations provides the most convincing support for our belief that high- and low-reactives possess differentially excitable circuits connecting the amygdala and the prefrontal cortex. These observations were made by Carl Schwartz, a psychiatrist at Massachusetts General Hospital who recorded the brain activity of our eighteen-year-old high- and low-reactive adolescents by placing them in a magnetic scanner. This machine allowed Schwartz to measure both the activity of the amygdala to unexpected events (as reflected in blood flow to this structure) and the anatomy of the prefrontal cortex.

The adolescents first saw a particular set of faces with neutral expressions, and then, unexpectedly, these faces were replaced with a different set of neutral faces. The high-reactive eighteen-year-olds showed greater activation of the amygdala to this unexpected event than did low-reactives. Recall that the high-reactive eleven- and fifteen-year-olds also had a larger waveform to the presentation of unfamiliar pictures. Similarly, a team of scientists at the University of Wisconsin found that young monkeys who possessed a highly excitable amygdala, along with high excitability in structures connected to the amygdala, grew up to be extremely timid adult animals.

The second observation refers to differences in the anatomy of a small part of the prefrontal cortex, an area with many distinct regions (figure 4). A small neuronal cluster in the medial portion of the prefrontal cortex, which sends impulses to the sympathetic nervous system, contributes to conscious feelings of tension or arousal that adolescents might interpret as anxiety or fear, especially if they believe they have just done something wrong. The eighteen-year-olds who had been high-reactive infants had a thicker cortex in this region on the right side, whereas the low-reactives had a thinner cortex in this location.

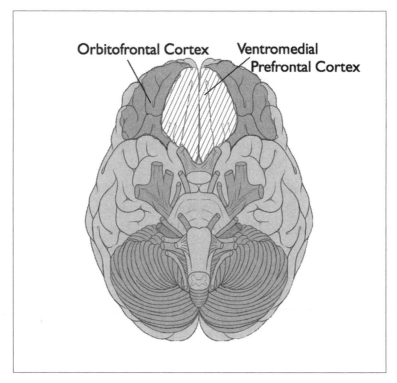

Figure 4. The underside of the human brain, illustrating the orbitofrontal cortex (shaded in gray) and the ventromedial prefrontal cortex (cross-hatched).

A second region, located on the underside of the prefrontal cortex (called the orbitofrontal cortex), sends fibers to a small cluster of neurons in the amygdala that inhibit the neurons responsible for the behavioral and biological signs of fear or anxiety. The high-reactives had a thinner cortex in this site on the left side; the low-reactives had a thicker cortex. About half of the high-reactives, but not a single low-reactive, had a thicker cortex in the medial site in the right hemisphere than in the orbitofrontal site in the left hemisphere.

The high-reactive youth with this anatomical pattern had been the most aroused, distressed infants and most likely to show arching of the back in response to unfamiliar stimuli. The medial area of the prefrontal cortex sends impulses to the neurons that mediate the arching response. These facts imply that the brains of high- and low-reactives may have been different at four months of age and biased the high-reactives to become fearful two-year-olds and anxious fifteen-year-olds. By contrast, the brains of the low-reactives biased them to become fearless one-year-olds and relaxed, happy-go-lucky adolescents. The low-reactives with a very thick cortex on the left side of the orbitofrontal area were among the small proportion of fourteen-month-olds who showed not one fear response to the seventeen different, unfamiliar events designed to evoke a cry or an avoidant reaction. These low-reactives described themselves at age fifteen as cheerful and were unusually sociable during the interview in their home. It may not be a coincidence that scientists at the University of Iowa discovered that, among a group of healthy boys aged seven to seventeen years, the youths who were most likely to be cautious and to reflect before acting resembled our high-reactive eighteen-year-olds in having more brain tissue in the medial portion of the prefrontal cortex in the right hemisphere. It is also relevant that a select cluster of neurons in the medial portion of the prefrontal cortex of monkeys becomes most active when an unwanted event occurs unexpectedly. Unexpected challenges or encounters with strangers are precisely the experiences that make high-reactive adolescents anxious. Patients with damage to the medial area, often resulting from a stroke or an accident, report fewer and less intense melancholic moods than those with an intact area.

What the Future Adult Might Be Like

All the evidence supports the claim that unexpected events, especially if they are unfamiliar, activate an already excitable amygdala in children and adolescents who were high-reactive infants and render them prone to anxiety in unfamiliar social situations. Intense anxiety with strangers or in large crowds, a profile that psychiatrists call social anxiety, is characteristic of about ten percent of adults in American and European societies, and high-reactives are at some risk for this diagnosis. One high-reactive boy, whom I shall call Frederick, was diagnosed with social anxiety disorder. This boy had been very fearful in his second year and screamed intensely when the woman dressed as a clown unexpectedly entered the playroom. Frederick missed many days during his senior year in high school because of intense social anxiety and feelings of panic in a crowd. However, rather than present the persona of a timid, quiet, conforming adolescent, which is expected for youth with this temperament, Frederick was an angry young man who peppered his answers to the interviewer with frequent obscenities and confessed that he had no hope of obtaining a happy adult life. Such a deeply depressed mood as

Frederick's was infrequent in this group of middle-class adolescents, but a psychiatric diagnosis of depression was more common among high- than low-reactive youths.

Although only 25 percent of the high- or low-reactive groups maintained the behavioral and physiological pattern that was expected for their temperament, very few children from either temperamental group developed a personality and biology that was characteristic of the other category. This outcome means that most high-reactives learned to cope with their tendencies to become extremely quiet and shy in unfamiliar settings. One such boy wrote an essay for one of his classes that described how he had learned to deal with his feelings: "I have found that the manifestation of my anxiety can be overcome by using mind over matter. I know how to deal with anxiety when it occurs. Because I now understand my predisposition toward anxiety, I can talk myself out of simple fears."

The most significant implication of a temperamental bias for high- or low-reactivity is that it prevents the development of the contrasting profile. That is, the probability that a high-reactive infant will not become a consistently exuberant, highly sociable, fearless child with a minimally excitable amygdala is very high— this prediction is correct for about 90 percent of high-reactives. However, the probability that these same infants will become extremely shy, fearful adolescents with a high heart rate, greater activity in the right frontal lobe, an excitable inferior colliculus, and a large waveform to unexpected pictures is much lower; only 20 percent of high-reactives met those criteria. Similarly, more than 90 percent of low-reactives neither were extremely shy or timid nor displayed several signs of amygdalar excitability, but only 40 percent were exuberant, sociable, and possessed signs of a minimally excitable amygdala. Only 8 percent of a group of boys from low-income families preserved a timid, shy personality from age two to age ten, whereas one-third of those who had been timid, shy two-year-olds had lost this trait by age ten.

Low-reactive infants are most likely to become the adolescents and adults that psychologists call resilient. These individuals are able to cope with poverty, parental or peer rejection, or serious mental illness in a parent because they can control the intensity of anxiety and anger that these conditions provoke. If they persevere and obtain a graduate or professional degree they often establish successful careers. Sherwin Nuland, a professor at the Yale University School of Medicine and a well-known writer, is a member of this resilient group. Nuland grew up in a poor family in New York City with a cruel, handicapped father who continually criticized his son with harsh rhetoric. But in a memoir written in his mature years, Nuland forgave his father for making his childhood so miserable.

A woman who had spent the first three years of her life as an orphan in the Nazi concentration camp at Terezin, but who had the good fortune of being sent to Anna Freud's center in rural England in 1945, provides an equally dramatic example of temperamental resilience. A psychologist interviewed this woman in 1979, when she was in her forties. The woman said she was a happy wife and mother and remembered, "I was a very determined child. ... I think I was very self-reliant.... I don't remember running to anybody." These adults are examples of the sanguine type, described in the second century by the physician Galen, who possess a biology that allows them to deal with life stresses that would impair most children with a high-reactive temperament.

The fact that a temperamental bias eliminates many more personality profiles than it determines also applies to a child's environment. If the only information that psychologists had about a group of one thousand children was that they were born to economically secure, well-educated, loving parents, these experts would be able to predict what these children would *not* become— criminals, school dropouts, drug addicts—but would have great difficulty predicting what they *would* become. The power of both temperamental biases and life experiences lies with their ability to reduce the likelihood of a number of possible profiles, not with their capacity to shape one particular personality. A temperamental bias resembles the inherited components of the song of a bird species. Although the bird's genes contribute to the basic components of the song, they do not determine the specific songs the adult bird will sing. That outcome depends on exposure to the songs of others and hearing its own sounds. Knowing that a bird is a finch rather than a meadowlark allows one to predict with great confidence the many songs that the bird will not sing, but that knowledge is insufficient to predict the particular song it will sing.

I confess to some sadness when I reflect on the fact that some adults, because of the temperament they inherited, find it difficult to experience on most days the relaxed feeling of happiness that a majority in our society believe is life's primary purpose. I have always wanted to believe that all individuals should be capable of feeling satisfied with their lives as long as they exploited their talents with care, perseverance, and integrity and established some close relationships. My understanding of fairness is violated if some adults who are idle and selfish feel happy much of the time, while some hardworking, empathic individuals are unable to achieve that state easily. If life were just, a high-reactive temperamental bias imposed on an innocent infant in a loving family should not make it so difficult for this person, who as an adult is prudent, persistent, loyal, and talented, to savor more well-earned moments of unrestrained joy.

Other Temperamental Types

High- and low-reactive are only two of a large number of biases that psychologists and psychiatrists have proposed. However, faith in the validity of these other temperaments depends on the evidence that scientists use to support their inferences. This last statement may seem pedantic or nitpicky, but I assure readers that such a criticism is unwarranted. Suppose that scientists wishing to discover the basic human diseases could choose from one of three sources of information gathered on 10,000 people: (1) their description of their symptoms, (2) analyses of their blood and urine samples, or (3) a CAT scan of their bodies. The first source of evidence would imply that headaches, stomachaches, muscle pain, chronic fatigue, sneezing, sore throats, and skin disturbances were the fundamental diseases. The second source of information would suggest that the basic diseases were defined by the presence of particular bacteria, viruses, abnormal numbers of white and red blood cells, or deviant concentrations of proteins or other chemicals. The third source of information would imply that the basic diseases were tumors, abnormally thin or clogged blood vessels, and broken bones. Each source of evidence would yield a different set of fundamental diseases. Fortunately, physicians are able to combine all three to arrive at a diagnosis.

Unfortunately, most psychologists and psychiatrists studying temperaments rely on only one source of evidence: parental descriptions of the behaviors of infants and young children (when studying childhood temperaments) or verbal answers to questionnaires given to adolescents and adults (when studying the temperaments of older individuals). As noted in chapter 1, most verbal descriptions are highly specific and not necessarily accurate sources of information on how the person behaves in the natural setting. Questionnaire evidence usually produces temperaments that differ from those inferred from watching children behave in a variety of situations. Several problems trail the sole reliance on parents' descriptions.

First, some parents are poor observers of their children and their descriptions are simply wrong. Second, the parents' judgment is colored by the comparison they use when deciding how irritable, active, or happy their infant is. A young mother with her first infant who has little experience with babies will be less accurate than an experienced mother who has had three children. Third, parents differ in how they interpret their child's behavior. For example, some mothers interpret their child's retreat when a stranger enters the room as a sign of "sensitivity" rather than fear. As a result, they deny that their child is timid with strangers when the question asked is "Is your child afraid of strangers?"

More important, the words in most languages, and especially English, are not always faithful to the details in the events they describe. Most words naming feelings and actions ignore the setting in which these events occur, fail to capture their changes over time, and do not describe blends of different feelings. For example, a woman who was robbed at midnight on a deserted street might have felt fear that she might be harmed, anger at the thief, guilt about deciding to walk home alone late at night, and sadness about losing her money. But if asked the next day what emotion she experienced, she would pick only one of those concepts. As a result, she might say she was afraid when, in fact, she felt a complex blend of emotions that occurred in a rapid sequence and were accompanied by different postures and facial expressions that were not available to consciousness. These are some reasons why there is generally a poor or very modest relation between what parents say about their child, or what children and adolescents say about themselves, on the one hand, and what psychologists and close friends observe or cameras record, on the other.

Many years ago my students and I studied a group of fourth-grade boys whose classmates agreed that they were seriously deficient in reading and unpopular, although all these boys denied both features when asked directly. We showed them a film of two boys their age competing in a cognitive task; one boy was described as poor in reading and unpopular and the other as both good in reading and popular. One-third of these academically failing, unpopular boys displayed signs of an emotional identification with the failing, unpopular actor in the film by cheering when he was correct or when the successful, popular actor failed. Thus, their verbal denial of their deficiencies was inconsistent with their less-conscious understanding of their talent and acceptability to others. Scientists interested in understanding any phenomenon resemble blind people, some with scissors and some with a jackknife, trying to separate an intact rose from the other parts of the plant. Each would come away with different parts of the flower, but all would be convinced that they had extracted a perfect example of a rose.

Mary Rothbart of the University of Oregon, who has spent years studying the temperaments of infants and children, relies primarily on parental descriptions derived from questionnaires. This information led Rothbart to suggest four basic temperaments, each regarded as a continuum from low to high frequency or intensity. Behavioral signs of fear, anger, or sadness, which Rothbart calls a bias for negative emotions, is one temperamental bias. A second, equally heterogeneous bias, which Rothbart calls surgency, is defined by smiling and babbling to events that evoke pleasure, along with a tendency to approach rather than avoid unfamiliar people, objects, and settings. There is, of course, some similarity between Rothbart's concept of negative emotionality and high-reactivity and between surgency and low-reactivity.

Rothbart's other two temperaments are less obviously related to high- or low-reactivity. One refers to infants who soothe easily, are extremely attentive, are able to control their emotions, and often fail to show signs of pleasure. The degree of regularity in the daily schedule of eating and sleeping is Rothbart's fourth temperament; some infants establish a regular rhythm early in the first year, whereas others do not. On reflection, it is reasonable that most mothers would be sensitive to the behaviors that define these four temperaments because they have implications for how easy or difficult it is to care for the infant. But the behaviors that affect the ease or difficulty of rearing an infant do not necessarily exhaust all the significant temperaments.

The other major candidates for human temperaments are based primarily on adult answers to questionnaires. Unfortunately, this evidence does not reveal temperaments. Adults' descriptions of their own feelings and behaviors represent complex combinations of their temperaments, life history, private interpretations of their behaviors and feelings, and their understanding of the traits that their society and the scientists administering the questionnaire regard as desirable or undesirable. A nice example of the dissociation between what people say, and presumably believe is true, and their brain state is seen in the difference between a person's subjective feeling and the brain's reaction to a painful source of heat applied to the arm. Although all the adults were told they would be receiving acupuncture that would reduce the pain of the heat, only some of them actually did receive the acupuncture; others did not. Everyone who thought they were receiving the acupuncture reported an equal reduction in felt pain, but only those who actually received the acupuncture showed less activation of the brain areas that mediate pain. The ancient Chinese physicians in the first century BCE who wrote a manual describing the way to administer acupuncture understood the importance of faith in its effectiveness, for they wrote that the patient must believe in the power of the procedure; otherwise it will not work. This experiment demonstrates the important point that the meaning of the word "pain" in the sentence "Intense heat applied to the skin causes pain" depends on whether the verbal report of a conscious perception or brain activity supplies the evidence. The same conclusion applies to the meaning of personality when questionnaires provide the evidence.

One group of American psychologists who use questionnaires to measure personality has suggested that there are five basic personality dimensions: extroversion, conscientiousness, agreeableness, openness to new ideas, and neuroticism. However, scientists who study other cultures often find more than five dimensions, and some differ from the five described above. If contemporary Americans were compared with the Athenians of 400 BCE, loyalty to the community would be a salient source of variation. If those same Americans were compared with seventeenth-century

New England Puritans, piety would represent a primary basis for human differences. The current list of five dimensions could be popular only in a society in which sociability, a work ethic, and tolerance—not loyalty to others, concern with the community, or religious zeal—were the traits critical for adaptation. An analysis of the 413 Chinese words used most often to describe human emotions and behaviors revealed that variation in selfishness, mood changes, and dependence on others were major personality traits. The variation in these three properties is missing from the list of five traits that American psychologists assume account for the important differences among humans.

It is also relevant that individuals vary in their interpretation of a question. For example, identical twins gave similar answers to the question "It is hard for me to start a conversation with strangers" but offered dissimilar answers to "I feel nervous if I have to meet a lot of people," even though psychologists would regard both questions as having a similar meaning.

In addition, most personality dimensions fall on a scale of good to bad with respect to the values of contemporary North Americans and Europeans. That is, a majority from these communities would say that it is good to be extroverted rather than introverted, conscientious rather than careless, agreeable rather than disagreeable, intellectually open to new ideas rather than inflexible, and free of anxiety rather than neurotic. Tibetan Buddhist monks might question the desirability of extroversion and orthodox Muslims would be skeptical of the desirability of being open to ideas that challenge the Qur'an and the existence of Allah. The dominant influence of the good-to-bad dimension in the words used to describe experience tempts some psychologists to ignore very important differences among people labeled good or bad. Murderers, neglectful parents, lazy students, careless accountants, cocaine addicts, prostitutes, and corrupt judges vary in many significant qualities.

The ambiguous meaning of questionnaire evidence is seen in the self-descriptions of adults from fifty-six different nations. The replies implied that Norwegians were the most extroverted, Austrians were the most open to new experiences, and Japanese were the least conscientious. Direct observations of the behaviors of these groups would lead to very different conclusions. The ambiguous meaning of a person's words is evident in a comment that the philosopher Ludwig Wittgenstein made to a relative as the philosopher lay dying. Wittgenstein was profoundly depressed and anxious his entire life, never put down roots in any one place, was estranged from his brother Paul, had three older brothers who committed suicide, and years earlier had written in a notebook that he could not imagine a future with any joy or friendship. He also had the blue eyes characteristic of high-reactives. Yet one of Wittgenstein's last comments before dying was: "Tell them I've had a wonderful life." This comment provides sufficient reason to question the meaning and accuracy of what people say about their moods or behaviors.

The answers to most personality questionnaires give information on three questions a neighbor might want to know about a person who recently moved into the neighborhood: How easy is it to interact with her? Does she meet her responsibilities with care? Will she entertain opinions that are inconsistent with her beliefs? These three relatively superficial properties ignore a large number of other traits. Among the ignored traits are the consistency between what people say to a stranger and their usual behavior; the capacities for and display of empathy, love, shame, and guilt;

the degree of identification with and loyalty to the values associated with their social categories; their level of trust or distrust in spouse, friend, or investment advisor; the capacity for sustained expenditure of physical energy; the intensity of motives for fame, power, or status; the degree of hostility toward authority; sexual orientation; strength of sexual desire; and the degree to which the individual's personality invites others to nurture or to defer to them. Many adolescents and adults who were high-reactive infants convey subtle signs of insecurity that invite the more confident low-reactives to support and nurture them. Almost all the major religious and philosophical traditions agree on the six virtues: courage, a sense of justice, a humane attitude toward others, moderation, wisdom, and an interest in the larger, spiritual significance of the routines of daily life. No popular personality questionnaire measures the variation in the commitment to each of these virtues.

Thus, the evidence from personality questionnaires does not come close to covering all that we need or want to know about individuals. The problem with most words and sentences is that they are indifferent to important differences among objects, events, or people given the same conceptual name. The statement "the garden is pretty" could apply to a small patch of lilacs in a backyard or an acre of diverse flowers in a well-kept public park. Similarly, the adjective "unhappy" could describe a child living in poverty with a single parent who was alcoholic or a child in an affluent, two-parent family who had no friends. Put simply, words do not always honor the details of what we perceive and feel. This critique of questionnaires and interviews should not be interpreted as meaning that we have not learned a great deal from this evidence. It does mean, however, that verbal descriptions of a person's moods and actions are unlikely to provide great insights into the temperamental biases of children or adults.

Whether the evidence comes from questionnaires or observations of adult behavior, the initial pattern of temperaments can be likened to the first stroke of blue paint on an empty canvas that became part of a seascape, or the first draft of this chapter, which was revised at least ten times, because neither the stroke of paint nor the first version of the chapter is recoverable from the final product. Every adult personality is a merger of a pattern of temperaments and a history of experiences in the person's family, culture, and historical time. These mergers are analogous to the biological mergers in animals and plants over eons. For example, chromosome number 2 in humans is a merger of two chimp chromosomes; the lichen on trees is a merger of algae (closer to plants) and fungi (closer to animals); and some of the genes in the cytoplasm of the cell represent a merger of the DNA of the host animal with the DNA of bacteria that had been trapped by the cell. The consequences of these purely accidental events were not predictable at the time of the merger. The same is true for the personalities of one thousand adults born with the same set of temperaments. No psychologist, no matter how sophisticated, who had complete knowledge of my genome and my infant temperamental biases, but nothing else, would be able to predict my profession, the research problems I pursued, the quality of my friendships, my income, the depth of my relationships with my wife and daughter, the ethical standards I honor, my politics, or the hopes and worries I bring to the breakfast table each day.

3

Experience and Inference

Each child is born with a profile of temperamental biases that creates a coherent pattern, as the profile of hair and eye color and shape of the eyes, nose, mouth, and chin create a coherent face. However, each temperamental profile creates only initial tendencies to be vocal or quiet, vigilant or relaxed, irritable or smiling, and energetic or lethargic with regard to particular events or situations. Parental behaviors, sibling rivalries, friendships, teacher attitudes, emotional identifications with family, ethnic class, religious or national categories, and even the size of the community during the childhood years combine with a host of chance events to sustain, or more often to alter, the relative strength and exact form of the traits the early biases produced. Change, not fixity, is the more significant principle in human development because, unlike gold atoms that resist change, the history of a life-form resembles the flow of a symphony whose chords change with time. Each person possesses the potential for a large number of feelings, thoughts, and behaviors. Each distinctive setting arranges this collection of properties into a particular hierarchy in which each property assumes a certain probability of occurring. For example, the likelihood of becoming quiet ascends in the hierarchy of high-reactive adolescents when they are with strangers, but this trait descends in the hierarchy when they are at home with family members. Of course, the individual's history of experiences can alter the hierarchy present during infancy, and the family is one source of important experiences.

Two Kinds of Parental Influence

Parents affect their children in two quite different ways. They praise and encourage or punish and discourage particular behaviors, motives, and values directly. In addition, each parent's personality, behaviors, and interests are influential because children's perceptions of their parents lead them to arrive at conclusions about themselves. I consider first the parental actions that directly strengthen or weaken the habits and moods that originated in the infant's temperament. Each parent possesses a private, and not completely conscious, image of the young adult they hope their child will become, and this image is usually different for sons and daughters. If the child's profile matches the parental hopes, the parent encourages these habits, or at least does not try to change them. Parents intervene, however, if the child's developmental path deviates too seriously from their conception of the perfect child.

I remember interviewing an extremely anxious young man enrolled in the Fels Institute's longitudinal study who had inherited a temperament similar to Marjorie's. The boy's father, an athletic coach at a local high school, was deeply frustrated by his son's lack of interest in contact sports. Rather than accept his son's preferences for reading, music, and chess, the father communicated his dissatisfaction directly and the boy concluded that his father disapproved of his identity. Failure to win a parent's affection and approval implies that the self must be flawed, and adolescents usually blame themselves, rather than the parent's unreasonable demands, for being unable to acquire the characteristics the parent admires. These mismatches between the traits that parents want and their perception of the child's personality usually produce troubled outcomes. Ingmar Bergman's 1978 film, *Autumn Sonata*, captured the blend of depression and anger in the adult daughter who could not meet her musically talented mother's expectations that she develop a distinguished musical career.

In addition, parents hold different views regarding the best way to socialize an infant who seems to be unusually sensitive, irritable, or frightened. Mothers are more likely than fathers to be responsible for the care of the infant. Mothers with infants possessing a temperament like Marjorie's, who sense that nature gave them a hypersensitive, irritable child, belong to one of two types. One type assumes she can help her child gain confidence by minimizing the child's distress and protecting him or her from frustration and fear. These mothers hover over their infant, rush to soothe any crying, and suppress urges to raise their voices or to express dissatisfaction when the infant spills food, breaks a glass, or plays with a sharp knife.

The second type of parent, holding a different philosophy, recognizes that the child will confront a competitive, challenging society in two decades and, therefore, takes the view that the infant must be toughened up in preparation for those stressful times. These mothers wait a few minutes before they minister to a crying infant and will raise their voices or chastise their one-year-old if he or she has violated a family rule. It turns out that the latter strategy is more effective for children with Marjorie's temperament. In our study, high-reactive two-year-olds with the second type of mother were less timid than those whose mothers were overly protective and reluctant to provoke fear in their hypersensitive infants.

A small number of infants, no more than 5 percent, are born with an uncommon temperament that combines frequent irritability with an inability to be soothed by parental embraces, kisses, and playful interactions. These infants frustrate the mother's need to believe that her care and love have the power to satisfy the infant. The mothers who fail to realize that the problem lies with the infant, rather than with their own adequacy, begin to question their ability to meet the expected responsibilities of the maternal role. This idea is threatening because most American mothers want to believe that their love can satisfy the needs of their infant. Initially they blame themselves for their infant's continued unhappiness. However, most humans cannot tolerate the corrosive feelings of guilt that accompany self-blame indefinitely, and many mothers eventually shift the blame to the child by assuming that their three-year-old possesses an inborn streak of stubborn anger. Once this flawed diagnosis takes hold, a reciprocal hostility between mother and child forms and the developmental outcome is usually disastrous if no benevolent changes intervene.

I remember a family with an extremely irritable infant and a mother who blamed herself initially, but turned against the child by his third birthday. This boy became a rebellious adolescent and an alienated adult, openly angry at a mother who reciprocated the hostility through an undisguised rejection of her adult son. This sad outcome might have been prevented, or at least muted, if the mother had realized that the infant's temperament was the source of the problem and that she had no reason to question the effectiveness of her love for the child. Many psychologists and psychiatrists who are friendly to the concept of attachment proposed by the British psychiatrist John Bowlby in the 1960s incorrectly assume that most of these poorly regulated infants had mothers whose insensitive care created an insecure attachment during infancy and a disturbed adult personality.

Identifications and Their Consequences

Although the parental treatment of the child continues to be important, by the fourth birthday children are aware of the physical and psychological features that they share with each parent and with others of their gender. A few years later they recognize their degree of similarity to those belonging to different social class, religious, and ethnic groups. As a result, children begin to identify with these people and groups, and these identifications have profound effects on later personality. The establishment of an identification requires that two conditions be met. First, the child has to recognize that he or she shares some distinctive features with another person or group. The more distinctive the features (that is, the feature is shared by a relatively small proportion of people), the greater is the potential for an identification. The second requirement is the experience of an emotion, usually a form of pride or shame, when a desirable or undesirable event occurs to the person or group with whom the child shares features. This phenomenon is called vicarious emotion. When both criteria are met we say that the person is identified with that individual or social category. Many people recognize that they share some features with another person or group, but fewer experience vicarious emotions. I share many features with "older white males," but 1 do not experience pride or shame when I learn that an eighty-year-old white male won a prize or was arrested for larceny. Individuals are most likely to experience a vicarious emotion when they believe that others will have thoughts about them that resemble the thoughts they have about the person or group with whom the individual is identified. Thus, I will feel some pride if an impartial committee reports that Harvard's psychology department is outstanding, but not when the newspaper reports that an eighty-year-old white man won an international prize.

Simply sharing the same name with someone eminent can be the basis of a vicarious emotion. My former colleague David McClelland confessed to a rush of pride as a child when he read the David and Goliath story and learned that he had the same first name as this biblical hero. Edward Said, a scholar who wrote about the contributions of Arabic cultures, experienced an uncomfortable tension over his ethnic identification because his first name had a European origin but his last name had Arabic roots. The philosopher Ludwig Wittgenstein, who was born in 1889 into a wealthy Viennese family when Austria was a powerful empire, had a strong identification with the category "European." When he learned while teaching in America that he had cancer, he told a friend, "I don't want to die in America. I am a European. I want to die in Europe."

Parents and Family Pedigree

The child's first, and often strongest, identifications are with the parents because children share more physical features and beliefs with one or both parents than with any other person. Therefore, the parents' personalities, interests, and talents have a profound influence on the child's development. Six-year-olds recognize that they have the same last name and might share freckles, a dimple, or the same hair and eye color. Moreover, relatives often tell children that they look or act just like one of their parents. Equally important, children sense, unconsciously, that they and their parents share a fundamental biology because their flesh originated in the bodies of their parents.

These ideas invite children to assume that they and their parents belong to a unique category. But five-year-olds have also learned that animals, plants, and objects belonging to the same category share both observable properties and less-obvious features. They know, for example, that all dogs have the capacity to become ill, to die, and to produce litters of puppies, even though a particular child may have never witnessed any of these characteristics in his or her own pet dog. The belief that things belonging to the same category can share features that cannot be seen tempts children to conclude that they probably possess some properties of one or both parents, even though they have no evidence to support that inference. A daughter with a mother who is extremely popular and knowledgeable will assume that she, too, possesses the potential to acquire these same admirable characteristics. That belief creates a pleasant feeling of pride and allows her to feel more confident. Of course, if a parent possesses the undesirable features of alcoholism, depression, or the inability to control temper outbursts, the child will be vulnerable to shame rather than pride and the identification with the parent will be debilitating rather than enhancing. I recall as a child being ashamed of my father's bent posture and need for a cane because of his crippling arthritis.

George Homans, who was a distinguished sociologist at Harvard University, confessed in a memoir that, as a ten-year-old, he was socially awkward, inept at baseball and football, had few friends, and a poor grade record. Homans said that he coped with his feelings of rejection, shame, and anxiety by reminding himself regularly that he must possess some admirable qualities because he could trace his family pedigree to John Adams, the second American president. Hence, he too must have inherited a potential for great accomplishments. Had Homans been unable to identify with a distinguished family pedigree, he might not have decided that he had the talent to become an accomplished social scientist.

If Lisa's family had lived in the same middle-class community but her father worked as an unskilled laborer and her mother cleaned homes, she would have recognized that her family enjoyed less respect than the families of her classmates, and the bubbly confidence she displayed as a child might have been subdued by the embarrassment that accompanied her identification with her family. If Marjorie's mother had been a respected pediatrician, her father the mayor, and their home one of the town's grandest, she might have concluded that she possessed some admirable qualities and her anxiety might have been muted by this reassuring inference.

People can easily determine whether they possess an identification with their family or another social category by recalling whether they felt a moment of pride or shame following a desirable or undesirable experience that occurred to a member (or to members) of the family or category. Americans who felt shame when television stations broadcast films of our soldiers torturing Iraqi prisoners were identified with their national category, as are those who feel pride when American athletes win a gold medal during the Olympics. Many American and Australian films evoke moments of shame in their audiences by depicting the unjust actions of the privileged white majority toward the slaves of the American South or the Aborigines. Identifications cannot be willed, for they develop outside the voluntary state of consciousness that controls most hours of every day.

Gender

Most boys and girls identify with their gender and feel obligated to adopt the characteristics that their culture regards as appropriate for males or females. They try to be the best member of their gender category, because children believe that each category of things has a best exemplar. There is a best puppy, a best milk shake, a best holiday, and a best friend. Many American girls have been socialized to believe that females should be physically attractive, maintain close friendships, and be kind to those in need. Boys, by contrast, feel a stronger obligation to be strong, courageous, in control of fear, and able to resist domination by peers. Each gender tries to avoid acquiring features inconsistent with their gender. A female college student babysitting our 3½-year-old daughter in 1958, before the women's movement and the increased number of female physicians, reported that our daughter was puzzled when the student said she was planning to be a doctor and declared, "You can't be a mother and a doctor." Few three-year-olds would be puzzled about that point today, because 50 percent of America's medical students are women.

Because most elementary classes in America are taught by women, young boys and girls unconsciously assume that school and its activities are more appropriate for females than for males. Hence, girls are more highly motivated in the early grades than boys. American children also assume that the objects of nature, such as lakes, plants, trees, and clouds, are symbolically feminine because they are passive and sources of beauty. By contrast, many manufactured objects used by both men and women, such as cars, trains, and airplanes, are regarded as masculine because they are active and possess a force. In *The Odyssey*, written more than 2,700 years ago, Homer treated the origin of the pink fingers of dawn as female but the destructive force of an earthquake as male. Even the first names that parents choose for their children are influenced by unconscious representations of the usual names given to sons and daughters. Parents are more likely to give their daughters first names with two or three syllables that end with the letters "a," "e," or "i" (for example, Sara, Rebecca, Vicki, Lisa, or Priscilla), and they more often give their sons names with one syllable that end in a consonant (Marc, Eric, Fred, Jack, or Ralph). Boys who have names that are sometimes given to girls, such as Dana or Joyce, are apt to question their masculinity.

Social Class and Ethnicity

The family's social class, which is correlated with ethnicity in American and European society, always exerts a powerful influence on children, because the families in every society vary in their possession of resources, real or symbolic, that the community evaluates as desirable. School-age children identify with their class category when they see that some families have valued features; they have nicer homes, command more respect, and behave as if they are entitled to privilege. The families with fewer of the desirable features experience a compromised sense of agency and have a tendency to defer to the former. The features that define the status gradient always depend on history and culture. The signs of status were land and livestock in Colonial New England, but in contemporary America vocation, education, and income are valued.

Why do humans establish these gradations of respectability? Monkeys and chimpanzees establish dominance hierarchies, but an animal's position in the hierarchy is based on size and strength in males, and on the status of one's mother and grandmother in females. It is easy to argue that strength has evolutionary advantages because a stronger male has greater access to females for mating. But strength is not a good predictor of more sexual experiences, a larger family, or a more successful adaptation in human societies. There is no evidence to indicate that physically stronger men are more likely to have a college degree, a challenging job, a six-figure income, or a more gratifying marriage.

One speculative explanation of the universal prevalence of status gradients is that the mutations that accompanied the evolution of modern humans were responsible for a number of unique psychological characteristics not present in chimpanzees. The habit of classifying things, events, people, and actions as superior and good, or inferior and bad, which is present in all four-year-olds, is one such feature. Initially, feelings of pleasure and pain are the primary bases for evaluating an experience as good or bad. However, as the years pass, kindness, love, honesty, laughter, education, talent, loyalty, material goods, and work with the mind are added to the definition of "good" in developed societies. Hence, those who possess these qualities tend to regard themselves, and are often regarded by others, as more potent than those with fewer such features. It is difficult to prevent the development of this typically unconscious idea. The sixteenth-century Scots passed a law prohibiting all those who were not nobles from wearing any silk apparel when in public. America in the 1830s was divided between a large number of poor immigrants from Ireland and Germany along with a less-well-educated indigenous population on the one hand and, on the other, an educated elite living on the east coast who regarded the former groups as dirty, wild, and unsophisticated. This class division was associated with a person's political affiliation (Democrat vs. Whig) and religion (Baptist or Methodist vs. Presbyterian or Episcopalian).

I recall an afternoon in a Shanghai hotel as a member of a delegation of psychologists in 1973 when Mao Tse-tung was premier of the People's Republic of China. We were meeting with a Chinese professor of psychology who told us that social class was the only important determinant of variation in talent and personality. One member of our group—I wish it had been me—challenged this opinion. "Since China is trying to become a classless society," she said, "when that goal is attained, you will have nothing to teach." The hapless professor, who did not know how to reply, was rescued by an older man who was our guide: "You do not understand," he said softly. "A society approaches classlessness; it never attains it."

Carl Jung's family was poorer than most in his neighborhood, but his father's position as a country parson allowed the family to enjoy considerable prestige in nineteenth-century Basel. Although Carl felt ashamed of his worn shoes and shabby clothes when he was a student at a wealthy private school in Zurich, his father's vocation permitted the boy to enjoy a measure of vicarious pride. Although Freud's family was wealthier than Jung's, Freud had identified with an ethnic-religious category that was the target of harsh anti-Semitic prejudice in nineteenth-century Austria. It is probably not a coincidence that the mature Freud wrote that societies harmed healthy growth by interfering with each individual's natural propensities, whereas Jung celebrated the benevolent functions of a society's values.

Several years ago I met a forty-year-old Polish journalist who grew up believing that both her parents were Catholic. When the mother confessed to her twenty-year-old daughter that she was Jewish and had converted to Catholicism during the Second World War, the daughter was propelled into a deep depression. This shocking piece of information meant that the young woman had suddenly become a member of an ethnic category that was a target of derision in her society. A graduate student whose parents were Mexican immigrants with little education chose for a thesis topic a highly technical problem in neuroscience for which he was not prepared, but one that enjoyed high respect in the academy. When I asked why he wanted to pursue a question that did not match his skills or earlier interests, he replied, "I have to do this in order to transcend my family background."

A small number of accomplished adults who maintained an identification with a poor or minority family continue to question their legitimacy, despite their enhanced status and celebrity. Frank Kermode, a respected writer and literary critic who was born into a poor English family, wrote that he always felt like "an outsider." John Updike, whose family had less status than many in the Pennsylvania town of his childhood, confessed that on occasion he felt so nervous when he met a Boston Brahman that his childhood stutter reappeared.

John Wideman provides a dramatic example of the power of an identification with a disadvantaged class and ethnic category.

Wideman grew up in Homewood, a poor African American ghetto in Pittsburgh, but his family's encouragement and a teacher's faith in his talents helped him attend college and become a respected professor and popular writer. However, Wideman wrote that he found it difficult to suppress the thought, which bubbled up each morning, that this was the day the world would discover that he was a fraud. George Homans, the Harvard sociologist who knew John Adams was part of his family tree, would not have had this distressing thought.

Although it is rare, a few college-age youth from low-status families whose academic record earns them admission to an elite college feel uncomfortable interacting with economically privileged peers. Because it seems irrational to decide consciously to transfer to a less elite college, these youth manage to get themselves expelled for poor grades or mischievous behavior. Some African American commentators have argued that many African American high school students have failing grades because they have equated a good academic record with being white. If they had achieved an excellent academic record they would possess a feature characteristic of the peers they disliked—remember the Polish journalist's distress when she discovered that her mother was Jewish.

Another important reason why class exerts a significant influence on a child's development is that parents who occupy positions of different status usually adopt different rearing strategies with their children. Middle-class parents are concerned primarily with losing status, and they socialize their children to conform to the mores of the majority society. In contemporary America this means compiling a good academic record, staying out of trouble, and trying to be distinguished in some way. The advertisements for automobiles in magazines read primarily by upper-middle-class adults imply that purchase of the touted automobile will allow the owner to feel "different" from others. The ads in magazines read by working-class adults emphasize that owning the automobile will allow them to feel similar to their friends.

Many, but fortunately not all, American parents who did not finish high school and have an annual income of less than $30,000 communicate to their children that they are destined to occupy a lower rank in society. These parents tend to be relatively permissive of aggression and dishonesty if they think these habits will be accompanied by a gain in money or friends, and they do not consistently encourage a good academic record because they do not believe that getting A's will benefit their child in the long run. This rearing strategy explains why class differences in academic achievement are pervasive across the developed world. About 15 percent of Americans, forty-five million, are classified as poor. The half-million six-year-olds from these poor families are four times more likely than middle-class children to begin the first grade with below-average reading and number skills, twice as likely to be diagnosed with a learning disability during the elementary grades, and more likely to drop out of formal schooling before high school graduation. The best predictor of the number of homicides in 2005 in ten large American cities was the proportion of residents in the neighborhood who had not graduated from high school.

Allied bombers destroyed most of Warsaw during the Second World War. When the Soviet Union occupied Poland in 1945, its officials implemented the Soviet philosophy of minimal class differences by forcing families differing in education to live in the same apartment buildings and requiring the children from different classes to attend the same schools. Despite similar residences, playgrounds, teachers, and classrooms, the children living with parents who had a college degree obtained a better grade record than those from families without any college background. Better-educated parents are more likely to read magazines and books and talk about politics and science at the dinner table. These experiences, combined with the insistence on school achievement, persuade middle-class children that intellectual accomplishment has value and will bring praise and affection.

I once studied the different rearing philosophies of middle- and working-class American parents by asking each mother to listen to a three-hundred-word essay describing both the advantages and the disadvantages of expressing a great deal of affection to young children. I then surprised the parents by asking them to remember as much of the essay as they could. Middle-class mothers recalled more sentences describing the sense of security and pleasure that children felt while being hugged and kissed. By contrast, the working-class mothers recalled more sentences stating that physical affection made children weak and compromised their ability to deal with life's hardships.

Parents occupying different ranks in the social gradient differ in their treatment of sons and daughters. Middle-class American parents strive for gender equality and do not insist that their daughters defer to boys, worry excessively over their sexual attractiveness, or suppress competitive wishes to be among the best in the class. Many working-class American parents assume that their daughter's opportunity to ascend in status depends upon marriage to a man with a steady job and a good income. This goal is more likely to be achieved if their daughter is sexually attractive. More than 80 percent of the parents who enroll their four- to six-year-old girls in beauty contests are working-class families on limited incomes who, nonetheless, may spend several thousand dollars for the costumes their children need to participate in these contests. Poor African American mothers without a husband who are responsible for the family's welfare tacitly communicate to their daughters that it is appropriate to defer to the sexual demands of boys in order to avoid confirming the stereotype of the dominating, emasculating African American woman. It is generally the case that female adolescents from poor American families of all ethnicities are less likely to use contraceptives or to insist that their partner wear a condom. Middle-class girls, who are more fearful of pregnancy, more often practice safe sex even if it is less pleasurable for them or the boy.

The treatment of sons also varies with class. Working-class parents encourage the acquisition of strength and sexual prowess; middle-class families encourage a gentler face in their sons because they want them to be accommodating toward the females they will court and marry. Thus, by early adolescence, the profiles of behaviors, talents, interests, and beliefs clearly distinguish boys and girls from different class backgrounds.

In sum, the parents' direct treatment of children, their usual behavior, and the child's identifications with family, ethnic, religious, and class categories combine to create different conceptions of self and its future opportunities. Because many adults who grew up in families occupying a lower status or belonging to a disadvantaged minority feel less secure about their futures, they are more likely to smoke, abuse alcohol or drugs, gain excessive weight, and experience depression, anger, or anxiety at levels that are more persistent than the levels created by the genes that contribute to these psychological features. A 1996 survey of Americans revealed that women from less-advantaged families reported the highest levels of anxiety, anger, and sadness. Less-well-educated adults are more likely to work at a job in which they are supervised by others. This situation creates anger, anxiety, or both during each workday. The persistence of this psychological state, which can alter gene and physiological functioning, contributes to the fact that most diseases are more prevalent and life expectancy shorter by several years in adults from lower social ranks, compared with those from higher-status groups. The life expectancy of British citizens in professional jobs is seven years longer than the life expectancy of unskilled workers—seventy-nine years vs. seventy-two years.

But a childhood of disadvantage, like a temperament, represents only an initial bias and does not determine the adult adjustment. Many children who grow up in poor or minority families become gratified, successful adults. This fact is the foundation of the American dream and the reason why so many poor immigrants leave their native land to find a better life in the United States. Neither temperaments nor the experiences linked to social class determine a person's future. Each is only a bias that can be overcome.

Analogous phenomena occur in monkeys, baboons, and chimpanzees, who form dominance hierarchies based on strength and boldness. The male monkeys that are dominant at a particular time secrete more sex hormone than those that are subordinate because they have to be ready to defend their high rank against those that challenge them. The subordinate monkeys secrete more of the stress hormone cortisol to a challenge and often groom the more dominant animals, presumably to curry favor with them. Among baboons, which usually live in groups of about one hundred individuals, each adult knows the rank of every other animal. The same is true for humans who interact regularly with about one hundred others. A species of fish living in the coral reefs of the Pacific Ocean provides an extraordinary example of the effects of social rank. Groups of six or seven females, which belong to a harem dominated by a male, form a hierarchy in which one female is dominant over the others. If the male dies or is killed by a predator the alpha female undergoes an anatomical and physiological transformation and becomes a male! The consequences of high or low status, in animals and humans, are among the most robust facts that social scientists have discovered.

Sibling Position

The number and spacing of older and younger siblings have a small, but detectable, influence on the child's attitudes, emotions, and behaviors. Helen Koch, a child psychologist who worked at the University of Chicago in the 1950s, studied five- and six-year-olds from intact, mainly middle-class families with two children. The firstborn, compared with later-born, children were more competitive, more upset when they lost a contest or received a poor grade, and more concerned with their status among peers.

Most firstborn, middle-class children who have affectionate parents find it easy to accept parental demands for school achievement and to view legitimate authorities—teachers, police, doctors—as desirable models to emulate. This favorable attitude toward authority is an extension of their perception of parents as caring, concerned with their welfare, and usually just when they dispense punishments. It is not surprising, therefore, that first-borns are overrepresented among each year's valedictorians at America's high schools and colleges and in the pages of *Who's*

Who in America. When two brothers were both major league baseball players, but neither a pitcher, the older brother usually had a higher batting average than the younger one.

Later-borns, especially if the interval between them and the next older sibling of the same gender is less than four years, envy what they perceive as the special attention and privileges the eldest receives and harbor a private anger toward parents, which later extends to all authority, for actions that they believe are unjust. Unlike firstborns, who place a halo on authority figures, later-borns regard those in authority as possessing "clay feet." Hence, they work a little less hard in school, and if they live in neighborhoods with temptations for asocial activity they are more likely to commit a crime. John Wideman was a firstborn, but his younger brother is serving life in a Pennsylvania prison for killing a man during an armed robbery. Firstborns more often choose the vocations favored by authority, such as law, medicine, and business. Later-borns are attracted to careers as writers and artists, who typically challenge the status quo.

I was teaching an undergraduate class the day that the Warren Commission issued its judgment that Lee Harvey Oswald acted alone when, in 1963, he shot John F. Kennedy; thus the rumors of a conspiracy were unfounded. I asked each student to scour the campus the next day and interview any undergraduate who knew about the Warren report, ask them if they thought that judgment was correct or a cover-up, and, finally, inquire about their ordinal position. More firstborn Harvard students, who trust authority, agreed with the decision. More later-borns, who are suspicious of authority, disagreed. I am true to my position as a firstborn, for I believed the Warren Commission report. The temperamental traits of Marjorie and Lisa were supported by their sibling positions. Marjorie, who worries about violating her family's values, is a firstborn; Lisa, who often challenges authority, is a later-born.

The firstborn typically receives a great deal of affection from the mother because this is her first child. As a result, the eldest more often establishes a coalition with the mother and the second-born forms a coalition with the father. In families with three or more children, the middle-born youth often have the most difficult time because the eldest and the youngest receive special parental attention for different reasons. Thus, it may not be surprising that adolescents with both an older and a younger sibling are more likely to engage in self-injurious behavior, such as cutting the wrists, than the first- or last-born in the family.

Frank Sulloway, a historian and psychologist at the University of California, discovered that later-born scientists were more likely than firstborns to invent and to support theories that were serious challenges to the opinions of older, respected scientists and incon-sistent with the beliefs held by a majority in the society. Copernicus and Darwin were later-borns who challenged the biblical account of the earth's position in the cosmos or the origin of humans, and a majority of the scholars who supported their ideas before they became widely accepted were also later-borns. Later-borns were almost twice as likely as firstborns, across twenty-eight revolutionary scientific ideas, to support the radical theory, and this readiness to adopt the position of rebel was stronger if the later-born came from a less-privileged family. A majority of the scholars who first supported Freud and formed the International Psychoanalytic Society early in the twentieth century were later-borns. The passionate promotion of a bold idea that challenges the beliefs of those in positions of legitimate authority is more likely if the rebels believe they have a right to question the status quo. This state of mind can be created in different ways. It can be the result of worldly success, a life of sacrifice for others, being loved by someone who is admired, or the belief that one has been a victim of injustice and unfair treatment. I suspect that this last mechanism is the most common among the later-borns who promote original but unpopular ideas.

Of course, many scientists who made original discoveries were firstborns—Einstein is one example. However, more physicists who accepted relativity theory when it was still controversial were later-born. Equally important, the public's values were not seriously threatened by the concepts of relativity theory, in part because it did not understand them. Nineteenth-century European society was threatened by Darwin's ideas.

Radical writing styles that break with traditional form or content often emerge in societies that are geographically close to a more successful or dominating society, a feature that is analogous to being a later-born. Ireland, which was invaded and dominated by England for more than one thousand years, was the childhood home of George Bernard Shaw, James Joyce, Dylan Thomas, and Samuel Beckett. All four challenged the preferred writing style of their generation and the dominant values of their society.

My younger brother, four years my junior and growing up in my shadow, resented the fact that his teachers were continually comparing my good grade record with his. In an attempt to find his distinctive identity, he chose law rather than science. He became very religious in his fourth decade and reminds me regularly of my error in remaining an atheist. I suspect that his late religious commitment served several functions, one of which was to allow him to feel morally superior to his wayward older brother.

Size of Community

About one of every two Americans lives in a large city. But, surprisingly, the number of men and women listed in *Who's Who in America* who spent their childhood years in small communities is greater than the number from large urban centers that have art and science museums, extensive libraries, major universities, and many opportunities for self-improvement by motivated youth. More than two-thirds of the twenty-two men regarded as the most eminent cosmologists of the twentieth century, including Fred Hoyle, James Peebles, and James Gunn, grew up in small communities, as did our most famous astronaut, John Glenn, and presidents Jimmy Carter, Richard Nixon, Ronald Reagan, and Bill Clinton.

An important reason for this counterintuitive fact is that children continually compare themselves with others of the same age in order to decide on their intellectual abilities, athletic talents, character, and attractiveness to others. Imagine a fourteen-year-old girl, Alice, who has always received excellent grades, possesses musical talent, and has many friends in her rural Illinois town of thirty thousand. Alice will know very few girls her age who have equivalent competences and will be tempted to conclude that she is exceptional. If Alice lived in Chicago she would be aware of many girls who were as talented or more talented than she, and she would be forced to conclude that she was not exceptionally smart or accomplished. The experiences that occur in large cities remind each individual that he or she is not particularly special. By contrast, a talented child in a small town with fewer children of equal skill develops an illusion of superiority and an enhanced self-confidence. This robust phenomenon has been labeled the "big fish in a little pond" effect.

The probability that a high school student will be chosen for an athletic team, the staff of the yearbook, or a class play, or will win a prize at a science fair is much higher for youth attending schools in small towns than it is for those living in large cities with high school populations of several thousand. Charles Misner, another eminent cosmologist, attended an elementary school in the small community of Jackson, Michigan, and in the seventh grade won a prize at a science fair. Youths from small towns are more sociable than those in large cities, encounter fewer strangers, and are less likely to feel the anonymity that can develop in cities of several million. That fact may explain why the incidence of mental disorders was a trifle lower among rural residents of England, Scotland, and Wales than among adults living in the large urban areas of these regions. Finally, adolescents in small towns realize that a majority of their friends and their parents would quickly learn of any asocial or mischievous act and gossip about their flawed character. This knowledge is chastening, and youth in small towns are better behaved than adolescents in large cities. The larger the community, the greater the probability that one will observe someone violating an ethical norm, such as vandalizing a building. As a result, the normal inhibition on the prohibited act is muted to some degree. For these reasons, two adolescents with exactly the same temperaments will establish different personalities and expectations of life success simply because they happened to be born in a small town or a large metropolis.

I grew up in a town in central New Jersey with fewer than twenty thousand residents in the 1930s and '40s and attended a high school with about eight hundred students. I was in several class plays and played the trumpet in the high school band. Because I had the reputation of being one of the three adolescents with the best academic records, the principal sent me to New York City to participate in a national youth conference on international relations. By chance, a reporter from the *New York Herald Tribune* assigned to the conference took my photograph, which was published the next day. It is a heady experience for a sixteen-year-old to have his picture, along with some celebratory sentences, appear in a major newspaper. This experience, which created an exaggerated illusion of superiority, might not have occurred if I had lived in New York, Chicago, or Los Angeles, where the probability of being selected to attend the conference would have been much lower.

Culture and History

The culture and the historical era within a culture set serious limits on the behaviors, values, concerns, and moods that are likely to emerge from a particular temperament because cultures differ in the profiles they praise, the ethical values they promote, the salient threats they pose, and the beliefs they hold. Consider, for example, seven major reasons for a sudden uncomfortable tension that a person might interpret as anxiety, shame, or guilt. Humans are most likely to be concerned with: (1) harm to their body as a result of illness, injury, or violent attack, (2) criticism from others for violation of a community norm, (3) coercion, domination, or intimidation, (4) loss of a gratifying personal relationship with a beloved person, (5) loss of property, (6) failure to meet a self-imposed ethical standard for achievement, friendships, or some other ethical imperative, and (7) uncertainty about the future. Contemporary North Americans, compared with those living in the same region in 1700, are less likely to worry about the first three reasons. As a result, the worries of items four through seven have become more salient.

The historical and cultural setting influences the hierarchy of concerns and ways to cope with the unpleasant feelings. The seven major sins in medieval European society were all private psychological states—pride, anger, envy, avarice, gluttony, lust, and sloth. An urge to yield to any of these desires would have provoked an uneasy feeling. In contemporary Europe only gluttony and sloth remain moral errors. The other five sins have been replaced with (1) failure to attain a career with high status and a good salary, (2) an unhappy marriage without sexual pleasure, and (3) lack of a reasonable number of close friends.

Individuals can reduce the intensity of the unpleasant emotion by commitment to a particular set of moral values; this strategy was favored by the Catholics of medieval Europe. A smaller number rely on the eminence of their family pedigree, as George Homans did. However, these two defenses have lost some of their earlier effectiveness and have been replaced by the possession of material wealth and a respected vocation. However, those last two strategies require individuals to compare their wealth or vocation with that of others in order to know if their status compares well. By contrast, one can recognize feelings of envy and lust without any such comparison. Thus, the unpleasant moods of modern adolescents and adults have become more dependent on the properties of others. In order to mute bouts of anxiety, shame, or guilt, individuals often have to persuade the self that its qualities are "superior" to many in their community. Had Marjorie been raised in a small village in France in 1200, she would have worried about her private sexual fantasies and her envy of and anger toward her bolder friends, and far less about meeting strangers, visiting a distant city, or failing to be admitted to a high-prestige college or university.

Seventeenth-century Europeans suffering from extreme guilt and depression believed the devil could occupy their soul and turn them into a melancholic witch. Contemporary Europeans with the same corrosive depression and guilt are apt to conclude that their mood is the result of a personal loss or failure to meet their high expectations. The historian Thomas Robisheaux described the anxiety that swept through the small German village of Hurden when the wife of the town's miller was accused of using witchcraft to poison a neighbor with cakes she had made to celebrate Shrove Tuesday in 1672. Contemporary residents of the same region would become angry upon learning that a chemical company's indifferent pollution of a local water supply had caused a large number of deadly cancers.

The poor Thai parents who sell their adolescent daughters to men who will force them into a life of prostitution provide another example of the influence of culture on mood and behavior. Thailand has an unusually large number of child prostitutes because of the high prevalence of poverty and a philosophy popular in northern Thailand, called Theravada Buddhism, which declares that daughters have an obligation to help their impoverished parents. If a life of prostitution is the only way to meet this obligation, the girl's behavior is regarded as ethically acceptable by the community. The prostitutes in Los Angeles who live alone in poverty engage in the same behavior in order to survive. For almost seven hundred years, from 400 to 1100 CE, a fair number of poor European parents killed infants they could not feed. Today, poor parents who cannot feed their infants place them with an agency for adoption.

Seventeenth-century parents in Colonial America imposed unusually stiff sanctions on children for displays of excessive autonomy or disobedience. Samuel Byrd punished a child dependent who had wet his bed by forcing him to drink "a pint of piss." Although Japanese fathers before the Second World War were unusually strict with their sons, many became accomplished professionals. The president of a successful automobile company recalled his father: "Once his anger was over he did not nag or complain, but when he was angry I was really afraid of him." An equally successful Japanese physician remembered, "My father was above all an awesome, frightening being. He was often enraged. ... When I overheard my father reprimanding somebody in the next room, a cold shiver used to run down my spine." These fathers did not believe they were rejecting parents, and their sons did not feel unloved, because a child's belief that he or she is loved or rejected by a parent is a private interpretation of the parent's behavior.

Most fourteenth-century European children were expected to be religious; contemporary European and American youth are able to decide whether they want to be religious, agnostic, or atheist. As a result, modern adolescents who choose to affiliate with a church, synagogue, or mosque do so for reasons different from those that were operative seven hundred years ago. Children with Marjorie's temperament are likely to affiliate with a religion because the spiritual commitment mutes some of their tension.

The eminent French writer André Maurois, who visited the United States in 1927 before the Great Depression and the Second World War, was surprised by the mood of optimism, confidence, and idealism, compared with the cynicism of his fellow Europeans. Had he visited America today, Maurois would have observed considerably more cynicism and a serious confusion over the values that must be honored. The questions that provoke the deepest brooding have changed over time. A thousand years ago Europeans wondered about what it meant to "know something." Seven hundred years later the concerns shifted to the qualities that defined human nature and the laws governing the universe. Many contemporary adults spend more moments than those who came before them wondering which ethical standards require reflex obedience.

Historical changes in population density have affected the vulnerability to feeling ashamed over an action. The decrease in the number of small villages and the sharp increase in the number of urban areas with more than 5 million people, some of whom have been residents for only a few years, have created large numbers of adolescents and adults who do not worry excessively over the opinions of the many strangers they meet each day. These changes imply that a temperament that rendered children susceptible to the facial flushing that accompanies embarrassment over violating a consensual norm has become a less important determinant of personality.

Finally, the historical era during which the child and adolescent years are spent affects the relative strengths of the child's identifications with family, ethnicity, religion, and nationality. For example, the residents of Colonial New England had more intense identifications with their ethnicity and nationality than with their social class, because the former categories contrasted with the large numbers of Indians in the region and the variation in wealth was modest. By 1890, however, industrialization had created a much larger gap in privilege between the affluent and the poor, and as a result, an identification with one's social class ascended in significance. Two decades later the Protestant majority felt threatened when the number of European immigrants with Catholic and Jewish backgrounds increased in a major way. As a result, an identification with one's religion became more salient than it had been one hundred years earlier when the diversity in religious commitment was much smaller. The extraordinary degree of ethnic and religious diversity in contemporary America implies that these categories engender more intense identifications than nationality for a large segment of the population. Such a situation makes it difficult for political leaders to rely on patriotism to solve a national crisis.

A chronic concern over possible betrayal by a lover, spouse, close friend, or employer has become an especially salient source of worry in contemporary America over the past fifty years. The popularity of the novel and film *The Kite Runner* and the songs that adolescents download most often reflect the ascendance of this psychological state as a function of historical events. One important condition, mentioned earlier, was the rise in the number of large urban areas containing migrants from small villages who did not know most of the individuals they met. A second, later contribution came from the writings of late-twentieth-century psychologists, biologists, and economists declaring, despite the absence of convincing evidence, that individuals were obeying natural law when they awarded greater prominence to their personal happiness than to the welfare of family and close friends. There is historical continuity from Adam Smith's eighteenth-century declaration that society would prosper if people pursued their own self-interest to the arguments of psychoanalysts, sociobiologists, and economists insisting that humans, like other animals, would be more content, more fit, and more rational if they first satisfied their desires before attending to the needs or expectations of others. Acceptance of this premise means that many individuals assume that their friend, lover, or spouse is prepared to betray them if they have to choose between their personal desires and those of others.

I suspect that the range of temperaments in Athens in 400 BCE was not very different from the range in contemporary Athens. However, contemporary social conditions have sculpted these biases into some personality types that Plato might not have recognized or understood, including adolescent girls who engage in binge eating and purging, wrist cutting, and oral sex and adolescent boys who use and sell cocaine and join gangs that engage in deadly rivalries with other groups in the city. That is why I suggested that temperaments do not determine the personality that emerges in adolescence; rather, they only limit the range of possibilities.

Let us assume that humans are capable of acquiring any one of two thousand unique profiles of abilities, motivations, values, and emotions. A particular temperament eliminates a large number of these two thousand possibilities, but a substantial number remain. The temperament Marjorie inherited made it unlikely that she would become a bold, sociable, extroverted, exuberant adolescent, but this bias did not preclude the possibility of a happy marriage, a satisfying motherhood, and an accomplished career as a writer. Lisa's profile made it unlikely that she would become a social phobic prone to depression, suicidal thoughts, and an aversion to risk. But Lisa might be unhappily married, disappointed in her child's school grades, and a frustrated professional.

A person asked to predict the exact place where a ten-pound rock that has begun to roll down a one thousand-foot mountain will eventually land can eliminate a large number of possible resting places simply by knowing the rock's weight, shape, and position at the top. However, prediction of the final resting place is impossible because the observer cannot know the gullies, stones, and branches the rock will strike on its long descent. A child's social class, ethnicity, and sibling position, as well as the experience of divorce, parental death, mental illness in a relative, frequent moves, size of community, and other chance events can alter the adult outcome of an early temperamental bias. Because none of these experiences can be predicted during the first year or two of life, it is not possible to know the kind of adult that will emerge from a particular temperamental profile. If the earth's crust in the region of contemporary northern Italy had not begun to move upward about 70 million years ago, there would be one continuous body of water rather than the separate Mediterranean and Black seas.

Life experiences exert their maximal power on the 80 percent of the children and youth whose values on a trait are not unusually deviant. It is possible, but considerably more difficult, to arrange experiences that seriously alter the properties of individuals who have more-extreme traits. For example, historical events over the past century have made it easier for American female adolescents to display aggressive behavior. Although some girls are aggressive, it is still true that repeated acts of extreme violence are far more common among males. Most children who spent their first three years in an uncaring institution, which happened to infants in Romanian orphanages, have scores on tests of language and social skills in the bottom 10 percent of the range of values. Although adoption by a loving family can produce profound improvements in both traits, most of these unfortunate children will always be a little below the norm on both competencies because they had been extremely deprived before benevolent experiences were first introduced into their lives. It is easy for family and school environments to create feelings of anxiety, guilt, or sadness. But environments need the help of temperamental biases to create the unusually corrosive emotions of a Martin Luther or a Sylvia Plath. The old adage "You can't make a silk purse from a sow's ear" captures this principle.

4

Temperament and Gender

Although most cultures, ancient as well as modern, assumed that the different biologies of males and females contributed to the moods, motives, and behaviors that distinguished between the sexes, a small group of educated adults in Europe and North America challenged that premise in the years following the end of the Second World War. Led initially led by Simone de Beauvoir in Europe and Betty Friedan in the United States, increasing numbers of women argued that there were no important biological differences between the sexes and the traits that differentiated males from females were stereotypes created by the society. Few scientists would deny the extraordinary power of culture and socialization to create distinctive profiles for each gender. The different traits of men and women in Saudi Arabia, Japan, Tanzania, Bolivia, and America affirm the power of culture.

Despite the obvious influences of culture and history, a small number of psychological characteristics do separate most males from most females across continents and millennia as a result of their distinctive biological makeup. Before speculating on these biological profiles, which represent temperamental profiles, I will summarize the research literature pointing to some of the psychological differences between the sexes that appear to be close to universal.

Psychological Differences between the Sexes

The sex differences observed during early childhood, before friends, teachers, and the media have had a major influence, are likely to reveal the more fundamental biases that each sex brings to the developmental journey. An important point to remember is that when scientists attribute a specific trait to one sex they mean that females and males differ in the frequency or intensity of the trait. They do not mean to imply that the trait is present in only one of the sexes.

Although scientists have not studied every culture and have little or no information on societies that have disappeared, the evidence supports the validity of a consistent set of differences between the sexes. Across most societies, boys (1) engage more often in vigorous activities involving the large muscles, (2) prefer competitive games with a winner and many losers, and (3) more frequently display physical aggression toward peers and acts of disobedience toward adults. By contrast, girls (1) play with a smaller number of same-sex peers in relationships that promote emotional closeness rather than competition, (2) show more intense and more frequent signs of fear or anxiety to poten-tial harm or social rejection, and (3) initially are advanced in language abilities.

More than fifty years ago the anthropologists John and Beatrice Whiting sent their students to a village or small town in each of six societies—the Philippines, Kenya, northern India, southern Mexico, the island of Okinawa, and New England—to observe the behaviors of four- to nine-year-old children in natural settings. What they found was not surprising. In almost every culture girls were more nurturing of others than boys; boys were more aggressive, hurled more insults, and engaged in more rough-and-tumble play than girls. Other research with American and European pre-adolescents affirms these behavioral differences. The dreams of boys have more aggressive than affiliative content; girls' dreams exhibit the opposite profile.

I have watched many two- and three-year-old boys and girls play in laboratory rooms containing toys and cabinets. About 20 percent of the boys opened the drawers of the large cabinets and crawled inside; I have never seen a girl use her body in that unusual way. When a pair of young girls who were strangers to each other met in a playroom it usually required only a few minutes before they began to play together cooperatively. A pair of boys remained wary of each other for much longer.

First-grade American children believe in a symbolic association between potency and maleness and between gentleness and femaleness. Children in one of my studies were shown pairs of pictures illustrating objects or animals that differed in strength, power, or timidity and pointed to the picture that was more like a man and the picture they believed was more like a woman. Most children selected the stronger, more powerful, and less fearful object or animal as symbolic of maleness and chose the less potent and more fearful object or animal as appropriate for females. For example, six-year-olds shown a large and a small table of the same shape and color pointed to the former as symbolizing a man. They also regarded a saw-toothed design as symbolic of maleness, and a curved design as symbolic of femaleness. When asked why, the children said that the angularity of the saw-toothed design implied a potential to cause harm. It is probably not a coincidence that Plato believed that the invisible forms (Plato's version of atoms) that made a food taste sour had an angular shape, resembling a saw-toothed design, but round forms produced sweet tastes.

Leslie Brody, who wrote an informative book on sex differences, cited a seven-year-old girl called Sophie who said, "I really don't want to be strong. I don't want to be big and have muscles," whereas a six-year-old boy noted, "If a girl was rough, nobody would play with her." Although the cognitive advances that accompany brain maturation make seven-year-old children more flexible in their stereotypes, girls of all ages have more freedom to adopt masculine traits than boys have for female characteristics. Boys who adopt characteristics that are inappropriate for their gender are more likely to be rejected by friends than girls who violate the stereotypes for their category.

Size and strength are salient qualities among all animals, including our species. All children recognize that, on average, boys are larger, stronger, and can run faster than girls. These initial perceptions are difficult to eradicate even though most American men have desk jobs and some women work on highway construction crews. Hence, children around the world agree with the ancient Greeks that males are more potent than females. (Aristotle believed that women and men made identical seeds to form the embryo. The female's seed was in her menses; the male's was in his semen. However, only males had enough body heat to transform their seed into the white liquid needed for reproduction. The female's contribution remained red because women had an insufficient supply of body heat.)

The symbols for male and female also apply to the contrast between natural and manufactured objects. Young children assume that many natural objects, such as clouds, lakes, and plants, are symbolic of femaleness, whereas more manufactured objects are symbolic of maleness. This bias has to be based, in part, on the child's understanding that only women conceive, birth, and nurse infants. During the nineteenth century, before the availability of reliable contraception, the capacity to conceive and give birth to an infant was the most salient feature of femaleness. Because the source of new life, whether a kitten from a cat, a flower from the earth, or a fish from the sea, was the essence of nature, it was inevitable that women would be regarded as closer to nature than men. And since reason was opposed to nature, Europeans attributed more rationality to males.

The wish to maintain harmonious relationships leads girls to be gentler with girls who happen to be unusually shy or fearful. Hence, as I noted temperamentally fearful girls find it easier to overcome their public posture of timidity. Unfortunately, most boys are harsh with frightened boys because that trait violates the sex role stereotype of a tough persona. As a consequence, very shy, timid boys become even more withdrawn. The imperative to be virile is a stronger cultural value among Latin American males than among American or European boys and men. The fear of not appearing to be "macho" with friends or women affects the quality of the Latin male's social relationships.

Most research with adults indicates that these differences between boys and girls persist. Adult men across most societies are more aggressive and make more attempts to dominate others. Women are more vulnerable to anxiety, depression, and feelings of disgust toward dirt, insects, and small animals that they believe cause disease. Adults from thirty-one societies more often assigned the adjectives "active," "aggressive," "reckless," and "ambitious" to males and more frequently assigned the terms "affectionate," "anxious," "depressed," "fearful," and "gentle" to females.

Parents shown a photo of an infant with an ambiguous facial expression ascribed anger to the face if they believed it was a boy, but attributed fear or sadness to the infant if they thought it was a girl. Another team of psychologists examined the answers that females and males gave to questions about the personal characteristics that permitted them to feel confident and self-assured. Women from 115 different groups comprising more than 32,000 individuals were more likely than men to say that their caring attitude, loyalty to others, and religiosity enhanced their good feelings about the self.

Galen, a famous second-century physician who wrote about human temperaments, assumed that females possessed a biology favorable to the qualities cold and moist, whereas men inherited a bias for the qualities hot and dry. Because the combination of cold and moist characterized the winter months when many become apathetic, Galen reasoned that women were temperamentally predisposed to moods of apathy and depression. This early intuition is validated by the fact that bouts of depression are more frequent in women of all cultures. The diary entries of seventeenth-century English and contemporary American and Islamic women contain many references to sadness and depression. Alice James, the younger sister of the philosopher William James and the writer Henry James, who suffered several serious attacks of depression in 1867 and 1868, assumed her melancholy was due to her temperament and noted in her diary, "As I lay prostrate after the storm with my mind ... I saw so distinctly that it was a fight simply between my body and my will, a battle in which the former was to be triumphant to the end."

Males appear to be more concerned with their relative power and dominance over others than with the depth or quality of their social relationships. Men are threatened by a challenge, imagined or real, to their potency, whether potency is defined as the ability to dominate others, physical strength, intellectual talent, athletic skill, sexual prowess, the absence of fear, or the capacity to defend the self against coercion or attack. Females are more often threatened by any dilution in the quality of their relationships with others. Moreover, men and women from diverse cultures interpret the sexual infidelity of a partner in slightly different ways, although both genders regard the infidelity as a betrayal. Men are bothered by the possibility that the woman may have found a more satisfying sexual partner, implying that they have become less potent as lovers. Women are threatened by the possibility that a dilution in the intensity of their partner's emotional bond to them will mean the loss of a supportive relationship.

Even when men and women have a similar biological reaction to a challenge, their psychological responses can differ. College-age men and women belonging to same-sex crew teams showed equivalent rises in the stress hormone cortisol before an upcoming competition. However, the men who showed unusually large increases in cortisol told an interviewer that they were eager to win in order to earn the respect of their peers. The women with equally large increases in the stress hormone said they wanted to win in order to strengthen their emotional bonds with teammates.

Both François Jacob and Rita Levi-Montalcini won a Nobel Prize in biology and each wrote a memoir. However, Jacob emphasized the solitary, competitive nature of laboratory research, whereas Levi-Montalcini emphasized her collegial relationships with other biologists.

I served on a large number of committees dealing with diverse issues when I was an active member of the Harvard faculty. When the committee was composed mainly of men, the first meeting or two would be devoted primarily to establishing a dominance hierarchy rather than attending to the issue at hand. When women were a majority, the committee turned immediately to the problem that had to be solved and tried to avoid provoking hard feelings among the members.

Charles Osgood and colleagues from the University of Illinois asked adults from a variety of cultures that spoke different languages to apply adjectives symbolizing the opposing concepts *strong vs. weak* and *active vs. passive* to a large number of names of familiar objects, animals, and social roles. Men and women more often assigned the words that implied strength and activity to masculine objects, animals, and social roles, such as the sun, a lion, or a marathon runner, but more often ascribed adjectives implying weakness and passivity to feminine objects, such as the moon, a rabbit, and an infant. The female figures in the poetry and plays of the Greek writer Sophocles, whose works were celebrated during the fifth century BCE, were portrayed as less able than males to control their strong emotions. For example, in describing Aphrodite, the goddess of love, Sophocles wrote, "She's madness, raving loose she's undiluted hot desire. She is wailing with pain, with sorrow, with rage, with fear." However, Eros, the god of love, was described as possessing a greater ability to control intense passion: "Eros, unconquered in combat! Leaps down upon the herds."

The possession of an unconscious association between nature and female implies that a society's conception of nature might influence its stereotypes for men and women. The Catholic citizens of medieval Europe regarded sexual desire as sinful but natural and attributed to women a carnality and capacity for evil that probably contributed to the fact that women were most often accused of being witches. However, five centuries later, when sexual desire and its gratification were treated as sources of health and vitality, the conception of women became more benevolent. This more favorable view of women, which emerged in eighteenth-century Europe, was accompanied by a view of nature as a source of grace and beauty rather than harshness and death.

Of course, the symbols associated with males or females tacitly assume a specific context. Women play dominant roles in a region of northeast Spain called Galicia because the society is matriarchal and women work long hours in the fields. When Galicians say that women are gentle, they are thinking of them as mothers and love objects; when they say women are powerful, they are referring to their manual work; and when they report that women are subjugated, they are imagining their relationships with men.

Many of the sex differences are influenced by the fact that boys and girls, men and women, interact with each other and each group compares its relative strengths, talents, intentions, and worries with those of the complementary gender. A majority of six-year-old girls have learned that boys are physically stronger, can run faster, and are less likely to cry when hurt than most girls. These observations lead girls to conclude that females are physically less powerful and more vulnerable to pain and to fear. If a society did not allow boys and girls to interact with each other for the first ten to twelve years of their lives, girls might be less likely to conclude that they were the weaker sex. Although the objective difference in physical strength and underlying biology would not have changed, the children's inferences regarding their relative potency would have been altered seriously. That is why Simone de Beauvoir wrote that the concepts of male and female were social constructions. Analogous phenomena occur in animals. Young male elephants become extremely violent following occasional surges in the male hormone, but the durations of these aggressive episodes are shortened if one or two older bull males are members of the group.

However, the suggestion that sex differences would be muted or absent if girls and boys interacted only with members of their own gender is not in accord with observations of monkeys and chimpanzees. Male rhesus monkeys, like young boys, prefer to play with toys that have wheels rather than with plush animals or dolls because the former allow them to use their muscles to make the toy move. Furthermore, the differences between male and female chimpanzees from eighteen different zoos are congruent with the gender differences in humans. The female chimps were less impulsive, less aggressive, more helpful, and gentler with other animals than the males. The males were more active, excitable, and dominating than females. The profile of sex differences in apes so closely resembles the pattern in humans that it is hard to reject the conclusion that there are inherited biological bases for some of the sex differences observed in humans.

Biology

Although the biological processes that contribute to the psychological differences between males and females are incompletely understood and, like temperamental biases, are affected by experience, a few conclusions seem relatively secure.

Male Variability

Perhaps the most robust fact is that the physical and physiological traits of males are more variable than those of females. There are more boys than girls who have either extremely high or extremely low scores on tests of most cognitive abilities and more boys than girls who are unusually tall or unusually short. These phenomena are partly due to the fact that females have two X chromosomes, whereas males have only one. Because one of the female's X chromosomes is inactive in one-half of her body cells (the X that is inactive in any one cell appears to be due to a random process), any allele on the X chromosome that disturbed normal development would be fully expressed in males but less fully expressed in females. This is probably one reason why the debilitating syndromes of autism and serious language or motor retardation, which appear early in childhood, are more prevalent in boys than girls, and why most diseases, with the obvious exception of disorders of the female reproductive system, are more frequent in men than women. The gene responsible for an enzyme (called MAO A) that reduces the concentration of three brain molecules affecting impulsive behavior is located on the X chromosome. Therefore, an allele that altered the normal activity of this enzyme would be present in all the neurons of the male brain but in only half of the neurons in the female brain. This could help explain why extremely impulsive behavior is more common in boys and men.

The Sex Hormones

The variation in the concentrations of the major sex hormones—testosterone for males and estrogen for females—and in their receptors influences a great many psychological functions. Only males secrete testosterone during the sixteen weeks from the second to the sixth month of gestation, soon after birth for a brief period, and at puberty, although older females do secrete small concentrations of male hormone. Females secrete estradiol, the most important member of the estrogen family, for a few months during their first year and again at puberty. Testosterone is the molecular source of bodily estrogen in both sexes and is required for the development of male genitals but not for the female's sexual anatomy.

One consequence of the surge in fetal testosterone in males is a slowing of the growth of the left hemisphere of the brain relative to the right. This anatomical fact is in accord with the fact that more males than females have a dominant right hemisphere and are left-handed—a ratio of about 1.2 left-handed males for every left-handed female. A more dominant right hemisphere should allow boys and men to perform at very high levels of competence on the psychological functions mediated by the right hemisphere, especially the nonverbal talents of spatial reasoning, musical composition, and painting. Students evaluated the beauty of unfamiliar paintings and photographs while their brain activity was being measured. Both genders showed greater activity in the parietal area when viewing the scenes that they regarded as beautiful compared with those that they perceived as less beautiful.

However, the beautiful scenes activated the parietal areas of both hemispheres in the female brains, but evoked far more activity in the right parietal area of male brains. This intriguing observation implies that the male brains were influenced primarily by the spatial relations among the objects in the scenes, whereas the female brains were affected by both the spatial relations and perhaps an implicit semantic naming of the objects in the scene. That more men than women have achieved eminence in geometry, musical composition, and painting is probably due in part to biological differences between the sexes that include a larger cortical surface in a part of the parietal lobe of the male's right hemisphere.

The presence of testosterone in the male fetus also leads to a slightly larger neuronal cluster in a small part of the hypothalamus (called the interstitial nucleus) that contributes to sexual arousal. Males have their first sexual experience earlier, have more sexual partners than females, and are more aroused by pictures of unclothed women than women are by images of naked men. Young men rated the sexual attractiveness of females possessing very feminine faces higher on days when their concentration of male hormone was higher than usual and showed a slight rise in male hormone after conversing for only five minutes with an attractive, unfamiliar woman. The song "There Is Nothing Like a Dame" from the musical *South Pacific* illustrated that fact.

Male hormone suppresses activity in circuits mediating anxiety and fear, and, surprisingly, inhibits the contraction of the muscles used in smiling. Males of every age, from childhood to old age, smile less frequently than females. This observation is probably due, in part, to the presence of male hormone. Because men smile less readily than women, adults of both sexes rate photographs of smiling male faces as less masculine than male faces without a smile. The small number of girls born with a disorder called congenital adrenal hyperplasia, about one in every fourteen thousand live births, had adrenal glands that secreted a higher concentration of a form of male hormone when they were fetuses. These girls engage in more masculine play as children and as adults are more practical, reliable, aggressive, and less avoidant of challenge than the average female.

A small number of children born as genetic males with an X and Y chromosome are raised as girls because of the female appearance of their genitals at birth. But the majority of these children develop a masculine identity during adolescence if they are administered male sex hormone. The rapid acquisition of a male identity, despite no change in their genitals, affirms the biological foundations of a masculine feeling tone.

Estrogen affects the brain in ways that differ from testosterone. Estrogen enhances the volume of two brain structures involved in remembering the past, and American females outperform males on tests of associative memory. Estrogen also renders girls and women more sensitive to pain, partly because female hormone dilutes the power of the brain's opioids to reduce the intensity of pain. This physiological state could contribute to the female's susceptibility to anxiety disorders and an avoidant behavioral style. However, estrogen seems to protect females from an early onset of schizophrenia; males show peak onset of this debilitating mental illness between fifteen and twenty years of age, whereas onset in females peaks between twenty and twenty-five years of age.

The two receptors for estrogen, called alpha and beta, often have opposite effects. Activation of the alpha receptor is more often accompanied by a feeling of uncertainty, whereas the beta receptor reduces this feeling. Estrogen may also be partly responsible for a woman's decision to dress more attractively on days when she is in mid-cycle and about to ovulate. This molecule also contributes to the higher incidence of autoimmune diseases in women compared with men, including diabetes, arthritis, and multiple sclerosis, because estrogen enhances the processes that lead to increased cortisol levels and a compromised immune system.

Of course, the differential secretion of male and female sex hormones at puberty strengthens the sex differences that existed during childhood and mediates sexual arousal. Women who are about to ovulate in the middle of the menstrual cycle secrete more estrogen than during other times in the cycle. This biological state is associated with more intense sexual desire and a higher probability of smiling when viewing photos of handsome, unclothed men. A man's skin secretes a molecule (called a pheromone) related to the male sex hormone that is likely to increase a woman's sexual arousal if she is with a man, even though most women cannot detect this molecule on the skin because of its low concentration.

Finger Ratio

The ratio of the lengths of the second and fourth fingers (the length of the index finger divided by the length of the ring finger and called the 2D:4D ratio) has a modest level of heritability and is a rough index of the amount of testosterone to which the male fetus was exposed. Boys and men have slightly smaller ratios than girls and women (usually a range of .91 to .96 for males compared with .97 to 1.0 for females). The prenatal secretion of male sex hormone lengthens the last section of the ring finger by a small amount, resulting in a slightly longer ring finger than index finger and, therefore, a lower 2D:4D ratio. A female fetus lying next to a twin brother is exposed to male hormone, as is a female fetus growing in a mother who is secreting this molecule. Both groups of females are likely to have a more masculine finger ratio. Comparable sex differences have been observed in the paws of mice, rats, and monkeys. It is intriguing that the sex difference in the ratio is smaller in a species of chimps, called bonobos, that is less aggressive, than the better-known and more widely studied species called Pan.

Even though the magnitude of the relation between the finger ratio and a variety of psychological traits is small in an absolute sense, it is consistent. Girls with a less-feminine, or masculine, ratio have a feminine identity but are more athletic than the average girl. School-age girls with a feminine ratio told to draw anything they wished usually drew flowers with pink colors; girls with a less-feminine ratio more often drew people or objects in darker colors. Young men with very masculine ratios have greater muscle strength when gripping an object, faster running speed, greater endurance, more sexual partners, and more often have a broad upper face, prominent jaw, and larger chin, compared with men who have feminine ratios. Male hormone affects the width of the upper face and the prominence of the chin because these bones have receptors for male hormone. Men with this facial profile who run for elected office more often defeat a rival with a narrower or rounder face and smaller chin. George W. Bush and Bill Clinton, who were elected president, possess both features; John McCain and John Edwards, who lost their bids, do not. School-age Swiss children were asked to pick the person, from paired photos of two candidates running against each other in a French election, who they wanted to be the captain of a boat they might take from Troy to Ithaca. Their selections matched the winner of the election 70 percent of the time. The men who work on the busy trading floors of large investment firms are under extraordinary pressure, for they must make decisions involving large amounts of money every few minutes. Those who earn their clients the most money have to be able to control their level of anxiety because intense anxiety can lead either to prolonged vacillation or to an impulsive decision. The men who were most successful in this stressful work setting had extremely masculine finger ratios, whereas the men who made less money had less-masculine or feminine ratios.

Boys with a feminine ratio have a greater interest in girls' activities than most boys. A very small number of adult men experience a disturbing inconsistency between their private bodily feelings and their assigned gender, called gender identity disorder. The even smaller number who request a surgical operation to become a woman often have a feminine ratio and may have inherited an allele in the gene responsible for the number of receptors for male hormone. For reasons that are not clear, there are more males than females with gender identity disorder. Despite the importance of the sex hormones, the psychological differences between the sexes are influenced by other molecules.

Oxytocin and Vasopressin

Oxytocin and vasopressin, secreted by the hypothalamus of both males and females, contribute to sex differences in feelings, emotions, and behaviors. The concentration of these molecules rises during sexual behavior to facilitate the emotional bonding between a male and a female in animals as well as humans. A clear example is found in the genetically related strains of a small rodent, the size of a mouse, called a vole. The males and females who belong to the strain called prairie voles remain relatively faithful to each other following an initial five or six hours of mating. The females and males belonging to the strains of montane or meadow voles do not form a stable pair bond despite many sexual encounters. The strain differences seem to be traceable to the fact that female prairie voles inherit an allele of the gene for the oxytocin receptor that leads to a denser distribution of receptors in a brain structure called the nucleus accumbens. The male prairie voles inherit an allele of the gene for one of the vasopressin receptors that leads to more receptors in a brain structure called the pallidum. The other vole strains inherit different alleles of these genes. Thus, the biological bases for the bonding of female to male appear to differ from those that bond male to female, even though both sexes experience the sensations of mating. Humans may resemble meadow voles more than prairie voles— more cultures have allowed multiple marriage partners than have required monogamy. Some American husbands, however, may possess one or more of the prairie vole alleles, since the wives of men with a particular allele for one of the three vasopressin receptors regarded their husbands as exceptionally loving and faithful.

Oxytocin activity is greater in females than males, due in part to the fact that estrogen enhances its activity. Oxytocin enhances the transmission of bodily activity to the medulla and, therefore, should increase the person's conscious awareness of changes in heart rate, blood pressure, and muscle tension. Mothers secrete oxytocin when nursing their infants, although the locations of the oxytocin receptors that mediate maternal behavior differ from those that are activated during sexual behavior. Oxytocin also facilitates the establishment of close emotional relationships with others. Hence, it is reasonable to expect that more females than males will be concerned with maintaining close friendships.

By contrast, vasopressin activity, which is enhanced by male sex hormone and is greater in boys and men, mutes fear, raises pain thresholds, and facilitates aggression in animals. The more frequent displays of physical aggression by boys and men could be due, in part, to their higher level of vasopressin activity. Surprisingly, men respond to the administration of vasopressin by furrowing the muscles of their forehead, a reaction often seen when one is puzzled or angry. Women given the same dose of vasopressin show increased activity in the muscles used in smiling.

Dopamine

Dopamine is a fifth molecule contributing to sex differences in behavior, motivation, and mood. Dopamine has a great many distinctive functions and at least six different types of receptors that mediate different psychological states. One state is the feeling of excitement, often interpreted as pleasure, when a desired but unlikely event is anticipated or actually occurs. Rats, for example, display increased dopamine to the unexpected appearance of a morsel of food, but not to the unanticipated occurrence of electric shock because neurons adjacent to the site where dopamine is synthesized suppress the release of dopamine. Humans show activation of the neurons that produce dopamine when they receive money they did not expect, but not when they are surprised by a loss of money.

As with vasopressin, men and women react differently to the same dose of a chemical (amphetamine) that raises brain dopamine levels. Men showed a larger increase in dopamine in the striatum (an area that contributes to feelings of pleasure) than women and reported a more intense feeling of excitement. This rise in dopamine was especially large for men who liked to experience novel events. Men also showed a larger increase in dopamine when they expected to taste a sweet substance but were actually given a placebo.

There are two possible reasons why men and women might differ in the magnitude of the increase in dopamine and the intensity of excitement while anticipating, or experiencing, an infrequent but desired event. First, the female brain binds dopamine to one of its receptors more effectively than the male brain does. Hence, some locations in the female brain have fewer unbound dopamine receptors ready to be activated. Second, estrogen dampens the activity of a molecule that absorbs dopamine from the synapses; hence, dopamine remains active for a slightly longer time in female brains than in male brains. Chronically high levels of dopamine are associated with more frequent spontaneous eyeblinks, and the average woman blinks more often than the average man. Third, in addition to being natural painkillers, opioids also enhance the secretion of dopamine to an unexpected reward and male sex hormone contributes to greater opioid activity. These facts invite an intriguing speculation.

If male brains have more "open" receptors for dopamine that are ready to be activated, the surge of dopamine that accompanies a surprising solution to a difficult problem, the unexpected opportunity for a favored activity, or the anticipation of a rare but pleasant experience will activate more dopamine neurons and, presumably, create a more intense feeling of pleasure in men than in women. The pleasure derived from eating chocolate provides an analogy. Eating chocolate is far more pleasant if individuals have not had chocolate for months than if they eat chocolate every day. Perhaps one reason why men are more likely than women to engage in novel, often risky, activities in which the probability of a pleasant outcome is uncertain, such as high-stakes gambling, sport parachuting, climbing glacier-covered mountains, drag racing, or promiscuous sexual behavior with partners they have just met, is that these activities are accompanied by a more intense feeling of excitement during the preparation and execution of the behaviors. Consciousness interprets this excited state as pleasant.

An imaginative study of pathological gamblers provided support for the claim that the addiction is maintained by larger than usual rises in dopamine when the men are engaged in this activity. These European scientists followed a group of addicted, as well as a group of non-pathological, male gamblers to a casino and measured changes in dopamine (by sampling their blood several times) while they played blackjack for high stakes. The addicted gamblers showed much larger rises in dopamine than the non-addicted men during the ninety minutes of play. Moreover, pathological gamblers who were given a drug that suppressed dopamine activity reported that gambling had lost much of its pleasure.

Parkinson's disease is caused by a loss of neurons in the sites that manufacture dopamine. These patients often report that they no longer experience pleasure from activities that used to be sources of joy. Moreover, young adults who developed Parkinson's disease later in life reported being depressed or tense many years before the symptoms appeared. All humans must manage a balance between the desire for new forms of pleasant excitement and the wish to control the unpleasant feeling of uncertainty. It is possible that the usual set point in this balance, which can be regarded as a temperamental bias, separates most males from most females.

Of course, there will be some males who prefer certainty to the risk of attaining a new pleasure and some females who prefer the pleasure of new experiences over the feeling of safety that accompanies avoiding danger or loss.

This discussion is relevant to the debates among the faculty and administration at many American universities about the fact that many more men than women pursue academic careers in physics and mathematics, despite no dearth of women in most of the other sciences. Although women represented close to 50 percent of those who earned Ph.D. and M.D. degrees in biology and medicine during the past few years, only 25 percent of women who received Ph.D. degrees in one of the sciences studied physics or mathematics. Some psychologists have argued that the villain is a cultural stereotype implying that males are inherently better at mathematics and physics. Faculty who held this dogmatic belief might exclude women from professorships in mathematics and the physical sciences and, at the same time, discourage college-age women from choosing these fields. There is some truth to this self-fulfilling prophecy. Young women who believe or are told that women are less talented in mathematics than men try less hard and attain lower scores on tests of this ability. And young men who are first reminded that males perform better on such tests actually get higher scores than men who did not have their consciousness raised on this issue. Such results illustrate that the person's beliefs about causes of differences in a skill do influence performance.

Whenever a scientist discovers a cognitive ability required for the mastery of mathematics or physics in which males outperform females, however, the talent turns out to be the ability to mentally manipulate the forms and spatial patterns of objects. Males are twice as likely as females to obtain scores that fall in the top 1 percent of the distribution of scores on these tests. These men usually have smaller, more masculine 2D:4D finger ratios and, presumably, a better-developed right hemisphere.

However, an exclusive focus on intellectual abilities as the main reason for the smaller proportion of women in professorial positions in mathematics and physics ignores the real possibility that men and women differ in their motivation to pursue careers in these fields. There are at least two reasons why females might have a muted interest in these specialties. First, most of the discoveries that are celebrated or awarded prizes in mathematics or physics, compared with those in the biological or social sciences, do not have obvious implications for improving society or alleviating human misery. Because women derive greater satisfaction from activities that have benevolent effects on others, mathematics and physics are inherently less appealing. Many of my female graduate students who were doing outstanding developmental research told me in their final year of training that they had decided to become clinical psychologists. When I asked why, they replied that the satisfaction they were deriving from their scientific research could not compete with a more urgent wish to be of use to others. Remember, across most of the world's societies women are regarded as more nurturing than men.

A second, more speculative reason has two components. First, the status hierarchy among the sciences is correlated with the difficulty of mastering content and the probability of making an original contribution. Mathematics and physics have always been regarded as the most difficult to understand and as domains in which a highly significant discovery is less likely than in biology or the social sciences. Mathematics and physics are the alpha departments in the university. Recall that males are more concerned than females with their potency and status in relation to their peers. Therefore, among youths interested in science, males should be more highly motivated to pick a discipline in which they could prove their superior mental capacities and, as a result, dominate those who selected easier disciplines. Put plainly, some men are drawn to the most difficult academic fields because mastering them permits the men to feel intellectually superior to their friends. The molecular biologist François Jacob once confessed to a nagging "fear of having no talent, of being good-for-nothing."

In addition, the probability of making a discovery with extraordinary implications for society, or a more profound understanding of a phenomenon, is much smaller in physics and mathematics than in biology. A scientist who achieved either goal would be acclaimed by colleagues and perhaps the wider society. Two examples are the discovery of the uniform temperature of the cosmos, which affirmed the speculative notion of the Big Bang origin of the universe, and the building of the first transistor. Both discoveries were made by a team of men who eventually were celebrated by their fellow scientists and the media.

If men have a more intense desire to prove their brilliance, as distinguished from a motive for fame, helping society, or adding to a corpus of knowledge, and male brains are prepared for a larger surge in dopamine activity (and a feeling of pleasure) as they persevere for years while anticipating a discovery with extraordinary significance, it follows that more men than women should select mathematics or physics as their vocation. This mechanism could explain the gender difference in professorships in these fields without any need to refer to sex differences in the intellectual capacities for significant achievements in these disciplines. Marie Curie, who discovered radium, and Margaret Geller, who uncovered profound insights about the cosmos, had the talents required for creative research in the physical sciences. Such women are not more frequent among females interested in science because a majority of young women do not experience the "high" that their male peers do while working in these disciplines.

Over the past forty-five years I have had lunches with Harvard undergraduates who were the sons and daughters of old friends. Four women from this large group chose physics or mathematics as their concentrations when they were sophomores. Although all four received A grades in their physics and mathematics courses and felt they understood all the material, all four decided in their junior or senior year to pursue a career in another field because they did not derive enough pleasure from these domains. One woman told me that the content was arcane and too far removed from people; a second confessed that she could not generate the level of passion that the men in her mathematics courses brought to their work. I suspect that many women possess the intellectual competences necessary for outstanding achievements in mathematics and physics, but the anticipated satisfaction that these disciplines promise is an equally relevant factor when eighteen-year-olds are deciding how to spend their lives.

Although females who have submitted research grants to the National Institutes of Health in the five years leading up to 2010 were just as likely as men to have their grants approved, the proportion of professors who apply for grants in molecular biology is five times higher among males than females. This fact implies that these talented women are less highly motivated to request a large amount of money for a time-consuming research project. One important reason is that many women have young children and want to devote some of their time and energy to their family.

Unfortunately, many scientists assume that sex differences in intellectual skills are more relevant than motivation because cognitive abilities are measured more easily than motivations. This unfortunate bias is reminiscent of the man looking for his car keys under a streetlight rather than in the dark field where he suspects he dropped them because it is easier to search a lit surface.

A Speculation on Temperament and Gender

The evidence invites the following admittedly speculative synthesis. Males and females appear to differ with respect to three questions that members of all cultures ask throughout history: How should I relate to others? What should my role be in heterosexual encounters? What should I worry about? Although there will always be individual exceptions, I suggest that more females than males are biased to establish egalitarian, emotionally close relationships with age mates, whereas more males have a stronger urge to assume a position of dominance with peers. More females regard sexual intimacies as opportunities to bind their partner to them by making the partner's experience as pleasurable as possible. More males are selfish and treat sexuality as a source of hedonic pleasure for themselves. Finally, more females are threatened by the loss of an emotionally close attachment, and more males are threatened by a challenge to their status and their capacity to command the respect of others. These differences can be regarded as temperamental biases because the sexes differ in many biological systems.

However, the culture and the historical era affect the personalities that emerge from these two patterns of temperament. The biological differences between the sexes are inserted into a social fabric and a historical era which lead boys and girls, men and women, to arrive at conclusions about themselves and their desires. It is unlikely that any eighteenth-century European woman would have asked her physician to insert a small bead into her labia or clitoris in order to feel increased sexual desire. Although infrequent, this practice has been increasing over the past fifty years. American women enjoyed a relatively unique position compared with women in most nineteenth-century societies. They had more dignity, their husbands awarded them more respect, they led or participated in reform movements against slavery, drinking, and prostitution, and they established many secular colleges, including Vassar, Smith, and Bryn Mawr, that limited matriculation to women. Centuries earlier, most women gained power and status by affiliating with potent men. Today, many women living in developed societies are able to attain both power and status through their own accomplishments.

The profound influence of culture on its conceptualization of females is seen in the stark contrast between two documents written more than four hundred years apart. The Catholic Church's view of women in the late fifteenth century is captured in a broadly disseminated German document, *The Malleus Maleficarum*, written to prove that witches existed and to provide ways to detect them. The authors argued that witches were usually females because women were too weak to suppress their carnal lust and yielded too easily to seduction by the devil. Hence, women were "a foe to friendship,.... a desirable calamity ... when a woman thinks alone, she thinks evil." Compare this unflattering description with the conception of women held by the twentieth-century German novelist Hermann Hesse, who had Goldmund say to his friend Narcissus, who lay dying in his arms, "But how will you die when your time comes, Narcissus, since you have no mother? Without a mother one cannot love. Without a mother one cannot die."

The events of the past century, which have produced technologies that have connected most humans and their institutions and created natural conditions that could lead to ecological disasters, may have set the stage for women to assume a more dominant position in all societies. Women worry more than men about the vitality and civility of their community and are better able to resist the haughty carriage of excessive ambition and arrogance that men find too easy to assume. Men who had been delinquent adolescents but developed a close romantic relationship with a law-abiding woman, compared with formerly delinquent males who had no such relationship, were far less likely to continue a criminal career. Lines from a song in the 1950 musical *Guys and Dolls* contain this homely truth: "If you see a slob get a good steady job and he smells of Vitalis and Barbasol/ call it dumb, call it clever/ but you can take odds forever/ that the guy's only doing it for some doll." Viewers of the final scene in Michelangelo Antonioni's 1960 film *L'Avventura*, in which Claudia forgives her carelessly disloyal lover for betraying her, will be tempted to assume that her love will reform his pathologically errant character. Some might amplify this idealistic hope with an image of the women of the world ascending to positions of high power to correct some of the tragic mistakes made by generations of ambitious men striving to prove their potency.

5

Temperament and Ethnicity

The suggestion that human populations who have remained in a particular region for thousands of years may possess some unique temperaments encounters considerably more resistance than the claim that males and females inherit different biases. The worry is that a bigot might evaluate one group's temperament as superior or inferior to that of another. Nonetheless, geneticists have confirmed that human groups who have remained isolated for hundreds of generations possess distinctive alleles, some of which influence the neurochemistry or anatomy that could mediate a temperamental bias.

Luca Cavalli-Sforza of Stanford University, an eminent scientist in this area of inquiry, discovered a surprisingly high correlation between the geographical distance separating two human groups and the magnitude of difference between their genomes. This claim is obviously valid for the many species of animals that occupy different niches around the world. Birds provide an example. The degree of difference between the birds of New

England and all other birds in physical appearance, typical song, usual behavior, and genes increases with their distance from New England. The birds of North Carolina differ just a little from those in New England; the birds of South America are more discrepant; the birds from Africa are maximally different.

The probability of a change in the prevalence of a gene within an isolated population increases with each successive generation, and the larger the number of generations the greater the genetic difference between this population and others. Similar changes occur in the language of a group that migrates from an original home to another area. For example, the word *rex*, which represented the concept of king in the ancient Italic language, became *rix* in the language of those who migrated west and invented Celtic. In only a thousand years the sentence from old English "Faeder ere thu the eart on heofonum, si thin mana gehalgod" became "Our Father, who art in heaven, blessed be Your name."

A game I used to play as an adolescent provides an analogy. Imagine fifteen individuals standing in a line. The person at one end whispers a sentence into the ear of the person next to him or her, who, in turn, whispers the message they think they heard to the person next to them. When the last person announces what he or she heard, the communication is usually different in meaning from the one whispered by the first person.

Modern humans originated in sub-Saharan Africa between one hundred thousand and two hundred thousand years ago and migrated first to the regions now called the Middle East. Then various groups split off from this population to settle India, western Europe, China, and finally North and South America (figure 5). Thus, humans had occupied most of the earth by around fifteen thousand years ago. It is also reasonable to assume that, until the easy availability of ship and plane travel, more than 90 percent of the humans living in Africa, Europe, the Middle East, Asia, North America, South America, Australia, and the islands of the Pacific mated with members of their local community or region for most of the last fifteen thousand years, or six hundred generations. It took fewer generations to evolve the tame dog from the Asian wolf that was its ancestor. Moreover, in only sixty-five generations a tame strain of rats was established from the more common wild strain that bites the humans who handle them. Thus, six hundred generations of isolated breeding was more than enough time to create distinct genomes among the human groups living in different parts of the world.

Isolated human populations differ in many genes. For example, Asians and Caucasians differ in the alleles that place a person at risk for several autoimmune diseases, such as rheumatoid arthritis, even though the symptoms of the illness are the same in both groups. A small group of Jews living in Spain and North Africa,

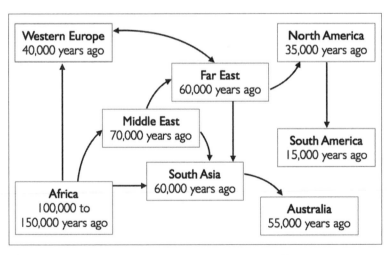

Figure 5. A schematic illustration of the estimated times of human migration from Africa to other parts of the world.

called Sephardic Jews, split off from the larger group and migrated between the sixth and ninth centuries to what are now the Baltic States, Poland, and Russia. The Sephardic Jews were joined later by those who were fleeing the Spanish Inquisition during the fifteenth century. In fewer than five centuries, and fewer than twenty generations of intergroup mating, these Jews, called Ashkenazis, acquired alleles for some diseases that are unique to this population, as well as some alleles that rendered them more vulnerable to one form of breast cancer. Ashkenazis are also less likely to become alcoholics because of an uncomfortable feeling they experience after only a few drinks due to the possession of an allele that limits the effectiveness of an enzyme that metabolizes alcohol. Biologists estimate that perhaps 90 percent of all American Jews can trace their pedigree to one of three hundred to four hundred families residing in eastern Europe five hundred years ago.

The Nature of the Genetic Changes

I noted in chapter 1 that genes belong to one of three types. Structural genes are the foundations of the proteins that make up human tissues and organs, but constitute a very small proportion of the total amount of DNA. Most DNA strings either control the expression of a structural gene (called promoters or enhancers) or are small islands of DNA within a structural gene (called introns) that are removed when a copy of the structural gene is transported from the nucleus to the cell's cytoplasm where proteins are synthesized. Many, but not all, of the genetic differences among isolated human groups are due to changes in promoter genes that influence the degree to which a structural gene will be expressed. Geneticists like to describe the effect of a gene or genes on a biological or behavioral outcome in terms of the amount of variation in a trait that the gene controls. The relation between IQ and grade point average in college may help readers understand this idea. The IQ scores of ten thousand college students explain only about 25 percent of the variation in their grade point averages. The degree of variation in the genomes of the individuals within a population is always greater than the variation between two isolated populations. Thus, the genetic variation among one thousand residents of Brazil is much greater than the variation between one thousand Brazilians and one thousand Swedes. Moreover, when scientists discover a relation between a gene and a psychological outcome, the amount of variation in the behavior that the gene accounts for is typically less than 10 percent. Although the variation in the incidence of lung cancer that is attributable to cigarette smoking is less than 2 percent, that does not mean that cigarette smoking is an unimportant risk condition for lung cancer. Thus, a gene that accounts for 10 percent of the variation in a trait is sufficient to create significant psychological differences between two human groups.

Gradients of Genetic Change

The genetic differences among the world's populations are associated with two geographical gradients. The east-west gradient implies large genetic differences between the residents of Ireland and those of Japan, because these populations were separated by mountains and large bodies of water that impeded migration.

The second gradient, which runs south to north, implies that the genomes of humans living in sub-Saharan Africa should be maximally different from those in northern Europe who were separated from Africans by both the Mediterranean Sea and the Alps. Even within Caucasian groups in Europe, there are genetic differences—between Finns and Italians, for example. Africans and European Caucasians differ in many genes, including those that affect the level of oxytocin and serotonin activity in the brain. African women, for example, have lower oxytocin levels than Caucasian women.

The proportion of individuals with the long allele in the promoter region of the gene for the serotonin transporter is highest among Africans (about 80 percent) and lowest among Japanese (about 20 percent), who are more likely to have the short allele. As a result, more Japanese should have lower overall levels of brain serotonin. This fact may explain why the Japanese who abuse amphetamines are more vulnerable to developing a psychosis than are Africans or Caucasians who abuse the same drug.

Latitude, which defines the south-north gradient, is correlated with the amount of daylight as well as the outside temperature during the seasons. These two conditions contributed to changes in the genes controlling the amount of skin pigmentation, body build, and briskness of the sympathetic nervous system. These changes helped adults living in northern latitudes adapt to the shorter hours of sunlight and the much colder temperatures. The paler skin allows individuals to absorb more sunlight, which, in turn, facilitates the production of vitamin D needed for bone growth. Adults who have always lived in northern latitudes (greater than 40 degrees and the approximate latitude of Boston) also possess alleles for one or more of the genes that influence the twenty-four-hour daily cycle from alert arousal to drowsy sleepiness, and the balance between the influences of the sympathetic and parasympathetic systems on heart rate and the arteries and capillaries in the cardiovascular network. The populations who have resided in colder regions for many generations have a more active sympathetic system. This system helps humans keep warm by retaining body heat through more efficient constriction of the capillaries in the skin. For example, the capillaries of Scandinavians lying in a bath of very cold water constricted a little faster than the capillaries of southern Europeans, and the capillaries of Africans required the longest time to constrict to the cold temperature. African American infants have a more variable heart rate than Caucasian and Asian infants, suggesting that their cardiovascular system is influenced more by the parasympathetic than the sympathetic system. Most of the low-reactive boys I described in chapter 2 also displayed a dominant parasympathetic influence on the heart, whereas the high-reactive boys possessed a more dominant sympathetic system.

Humans from northern latitudes are more vulnerable to multiple sclerosis and depression, and they find it easier to detect variations in shades of purple (short wavelength) than in shades of green (longer wavelength). Latitude has similar effects on animals. Modern domesticated cats evolved from a species that first appeared in Asia many thousands of years ago. The Norwegian Forest cats of northern Europe underwent genetic changes that created a higher internal body temperature than the temperature of the Siamese cats that live in the warm climate of Thailand. Bird species from northern latitudes have higher metabolic rates compared with related species normally residing in warmer climates.

Anthropologists have speculated that the physiologies that would be most adaptive in Africa would favor immunity against malaria and skin infections, the ability to keep the body cool, and the capacity to digest fruits and dense carbohydrates. The anatomy and physiology that would be adaptive in Europe and Asia, when humans were domesticating plants and animals and establishing relatively permanent villages, would favor the ability to keep the body warm during winter and to digest cereals and the milk of goats and cows. Some of the genes that contributed to these adaptations might have implications for temperamental biases. Of course, some genetic changes are the result of random processes, called genetic drift, that are not selected as advantageous or contributing to fitness.

Asians and European-Caucasians

Comparisons of the psychological and biological differences between Asians, primarily those living in China or Japan, and Caucasians living in Europe and North America have been explored more extensively than other comparisons. Asians and Caucasians differ in about one of every four genes located in the promoter regions that control the expression of structural genes. A critical question, however, is whether these genetic differences affect any behaviors, beliefs, or emotions. The answer appears to be yes. Alcoholism, for example, is far less frequent among Asians than among Caucasians because Asians inherit alleles that interfere with the liver's metabolism of alcohol and, as a result, excessive drinking leads to physical discomfort.

Richard Nisbett and his colleagues at the University of Michigan have found that Asians are unusually sensitive to and conscious of the setting in which a person behaves or the context in which an object appears. More paintings and photographs by Asian artists, compared with European artists, depict many objects, plants, or animals in the backgrounds of scenes that illustrate a central object. By contrast, European and American artists place a person, animal, or object of significance in the foreground and add fewer other objects. Asian American and European American college students without any special artistic talent displayed a similar bias when asked to draw a landscape.

When American and Japanese students indicated their preferences among a set of portraits that varied in the number of background objects, more Japanese than Americans preferred scenes in which the central figure was both smaller and in the background of a setting that contained other objects. The films made by Asian directors contain many scenes in which the central character is just perceptible in the background of a street, field, or home. Hollywood directors rarely film such scenes and prefer to present viewers with close-ups of faces that fill the screen. The Western preference for attending to the single focal object is even reflected in a viewer's rapid and unconscious eye movements across the elements of a picture. Americans were more likely than Chinese to focus on the central object and ignore the elements in the background, whereas Chinese viewers directed more attention to the objects or people in the background, although not ignoring the central figure.

The relation between self and the outside world also differentiates Asians from the Caucasians living in Europe and North America. Ever since the ancient Greeks, later western societies have chosen to make each person's skills, beliefs, values, and feelings the primary features of their identity. This emphasis on the solitary individual acting alone was enhanced by the introduction of Christianity, which made each person's faith in God and loyalty to a set of ethical standards essential for a feeling of virtue. These are the cultural conditions under which a "man for all seasons"—Thomas More, for example—is likely to emerge. The eighteenth-century German philosopher Immanuel Kant captured the European celebration of the self-sufficient individual when he wrote that a person who had no need of society would enjoy an emotion bordering on the sublime.

The Chinese, for an equally long time, chose to make each person's social roles and obligations to others the core features of a self. Loyalty to family, friends, nation, and employer took precedence over private wishes. A martyr willing to oppose the beliefs of the majority in order to be true to his or her own ethics is less likely to emerge in these cultures. The premise that an essential feature of humanity is membership in a community is seen in the fact that the Chinese used to punish a criminal by isolating him from all human contact at the bottom of a deep well. Europeans chose hanging, stoning, or a firing squad. The Japanese concept of *amae* refers to a set of mutual obligations between one person in need of help and another who accepts the obligation to support the supplicant. This concept, which can refer to a relationship between a teacher and a student or a supervisor and a subordinate, has no counterpart in English. The Chinese living in Hong Kong use the word *tongzhi* to refer to any person who is loyal to the ethical values of a particular group, independent of the content of those values. English, which does not have such a term, contains words that name the content of the values (e.g., "liberal," "evangelical").

Chinese and Japanese parents socialize their children to be hypersensitive to the thoughts of the people with whom they are interacting and the setting in which the interaction occurs. The acute awareness of others and the irrepressible wish to avoid upsetting, angering, or embarrassing them finds expression in the contrasting Japanese terms *honne* and *tatemae*. *Honne* refers to a person's inner feelings that can be expressed with intimates; *tatemae* refers to the face that is shown to the world. A close Japanese friend once gave me a classic example of *tatemae*: "Imagine you are sitting next to a stranger on an airplane and writing with a pen on a pad of paper. The stranger asks, 'What is that you are writing with?' If you wish to honor the obligations of *tatemae* you should not imply that the stranger did not know what a pen looks like; hence you should reply, 'It's a pen, isn't it?'"

The salience of the difference between the mental sets of *tatemae* and *honne* has influenced Japanese artists. I remember visiting an art museum in Tokyo many years ago and being surprised by the large number of paintings in which this contrast was the central theme. For example, one canvas of a pair of flying geese illustrated one bird with its feet visible and the other with them hidden. Another depicted two people; one facing forward and the other facing away from the viewer. European artists rarely made the contrast between what is visible and what is hidden the primary idea in their paintings.

Europeans and Americans are socialized to be true to their private consciences and not to worry excessively about what others think. A person would be criticized as a hypocrite if the character traits and opinions displayed at home did not carry over to the workplace or to a dinner party. Asians understand that a person need not be consistent across settings because one's role often varies with the context. A woman is a mother at home, a professional at work, a guest at a party. Put a bit too plainly, Europeans and Americans see each person as a well-defined entity with fixed traits acting on others in the world. Asians regard a person as a collection of distinct roles that are altered to fit a specific group of individuals who are continually evaluating the adequacy of the individual's performance. A person's qualities are expected to vary with the groups in which he or she participates, just as the meaning of a word often depends on the paragraph in which it appears.

The vulnerability to a feeling of shame if the person fails to display the prescribed role properly is one reason why public displays of anxiety or depression carry more stigma among Chinese and Japanese populations and why Asian Americans under stress are more reluctant than European Americans to ask their friends for emotional support. Asian children and youth experience distress if they believe they did something that shamed their family. American and European children feel distressed if they fail to achieve a desired goal, because the failure implies they have violated a private ethical standard. Although these differences are in accord with the distinctive socializations of Asian compared with European or American children, the possibility also exists that genetic differences between these populations make a small contribution to this intriguing variation.

The Role of Temperament

One admittedly speculative suggestion rests on the assumption that more Caucasians than Asians possess temperamental biases that render the former more vulnerable to frequent changes in bodily sensations that pierce consciousness and recruit attention to the self and its feeling tone. As a result, it might be easier for Caucasian American and European parents to persuade their children to be loyal to their private conscience in order to avoid the unpleasant feelings that accompany guilt over ethical violations and easier for Asian parents to socialize their children to be sensitive to others. Although there is no firm support for this speculation, it is not beyond credibility in light of the known biological differences between the two populations.

Behaviors suggestive of different temperamental biases in Asians and Caucasians can be seen during the early days and weeks of life. A pair of scientists discovered that newborn Asian American infants living in California, compared with Caucasian Americans from the same region, were calmer, were less likely to struggle to remove a cloth from their face, and were consoled more easily when they cried. Japanese infants, too, were less likely than Caucasian Americans to cry during a pediatric examination or inoculation.

You will recall that Richard Kearsley, Philip Zelazo, and I observed Chinese American and Caucasian infants, attending a day care center or raised only at home. The Chinese infants, whether they attended the center or not, were distinctly different from the Caucasians living in the same neighborhood. The Chinese infants smiled, laughed, and babbled less often, as toddlers stayed closer to their mothers in an unfamiliar room containing children they did not know, and displayed a remarkably stable heart rate.

Some of my colleagues administered the same battery of unfamiliar stimuli given to the large group of Boston Caucasian infants I described in chapter 2 to four-month-old Caucasian infants born in Dublin and Chinese infants born in Beijing. The Caucasian infants, whether from Boston or Dublin, thrashed their limbs and cried more frequently than the Chinese infants. Caucasian infants appear to be more labile and more easily excited than Chinese.

Although the low levels of motor arousal and infrequent crying among Chinese infants make them appear similar to the low-reactive Boston and Dublin infants, it is likely that the genes mediating the lower behavioral arousal are not the same in Chinese and Caucasian infants. The differences in ease of arousal to unexpected or unfamiliar experiences are retained as children develop. Chinese mothers in Shanghai described their six- and seven-year-olds as less active, less impulsive, and more controlled than did Caucasian American mothers from the Pacific Northwest asked to describe their children. In older children, Thai parents were concerned about their child's low energy level, whereas Caucasian parents worried about their child's aggressiveness and hyperactivity. It is relevant that Asian American psychiatric patients suffering from an anxiety or depressive disorder require a lower dose of therapeutic drugs than Caucasian patients in the same region reporting the same symptoms. This fact implies that anxious Asians may be at a lower level of limbic arousal than anxious Caucasians.

Recall that Asians differ from Caucasians in about 25 percent of the genes located in the promoter regions. One of these alleles controls the expression of the structural gene that is the foundation of a molecule (called the serotonin transporter) that absorbs serotonin from the synapses between neurons. Asians are more likely than other populations to possess an allele, called the short allele, that reduces the level of expression of this gene. As a result, there is less transporter, and serotonin remains in the synapses for a slightly longer time. Scientists believe that the prolonged presence of serotonin leads in time to lower chronic levels of serotonin activity in Asian brains compared with Caucasian or African brains. This outcome could occur if the excess serotonin in the synapses was accompanied by a reduction in the number of receptors for serotonin in the adjacent neurons. Lower levels of serotonin activity could also be the result of an inhibitory feedback loop from serotonin neurons to the raphe nucleus, the site that manufactures serotonin. This process would lead to reduced secretion of serotonin. Either mechanism would lead to chronically lower levels of serotonin activity, which would have a number of consequences.

Serotonin contributes to behavioral signs of pleasure, such as smiling, laughing, and vocalizing; hence, the higher incidence of the short allele among Asians might help explain why Chinese children smiled and laughed less frequently than Caucasians of the same age, social class, and geographic region. In addition, serotonin activates a specific dopamine receptor in sites that mediate limb movement. Thus, the low levels of limb movement shown by Asian 4-month-olds in response to new sights and sounds might be due, in part, to the possession of the short allele, which lowers the tonic level of brain serotonin and leads, in turn, to reduced activation of the dopamine receptors in sites responsible for bodily activity.

Possession of the short allele might also affect social behavior. Monkeys with the short allele are more vigilant to pictures of high-status male monkeys, and humans with the short allele display a greater brain response to faces with an angry expression. These facts imply that carriers of the short allele might be unusually sensitive to the signs of potential threat posed by other members of their species. Such individuals should be biased to be submissive (if a monkey) and conforming to group norms (if a human). This scattered collection of diverse observations can be arranged to create an interpretation that reads like a pretty story; I hope it has some measure of truth.

Geographically separated human populations also differ in the shape of the face. Asians have the flattest faces; that is, the forehead, jaw, and nasal protuberance are less prominent than those of most Caucasians and Africans. When biologists bred a small number of tame silver foxes (from a larger group of untamed foxes) with other tame animals, it took fewer than twenty generations to produce all tame offspring. These tame animals had less activity in the brain circuits that produce the stress hormone cortisol, developed fearful reactions to novel locations later in infancy, had small white patches of fur that were free of melanin, and possessed shorter snouts—that is, flatter faces. Many domesticated mammals that are bred to be tame, including horses, sheep, pigs, and cows, show similar features, especially less fear, less aggression, and shorter snouts than their untamed, wild relatives. The fact that the average Asian has a flatter face than the average Caucasian or African provokes the speculation that, from a biological perspective, Asians may be biased to be "tamer"—that is, gentler with others. Even Hippocrates, writing in the fourth century before the modern era, suggested that the people living far to the east of Athens were gentler than his fellow Greeks. It may not be a coincidence, therefore, that loyalty to one's family and social groups is a cardinal Asian value.

These observations imply that the genes that contribute to a tame temperament in mammals may also affect the cells that produce melanin in the skin, the differential activity of the sympathetic and parasympathetic systems, and the bone structure of the face. Can we explain this odd combination of behavior and biology? A small necklace of cells, called the neural crest, forms within the first weeks after conception, and different clusters of neural crest cells subsequently migrate to become the bones of the face, the pigment cells of the hair, skin, and iris, and the sympathetic and parasympathetic nervous systems, which control heart rate.

These facts suggest, but obviously do not prove, that the genes controlling the chemistry of the neural crest cells make a small contribution to the different behavioral and anatomical profiles of Asians, Caucasians, and Africans. Serotonin is one of the molecules affecting the differentiation and migration of the neural crest cells. Because more Asians than Caucasians and Africans possess the short allele in the promoter region of the gene responsible for the serotonin transporter, it is possible that one small basis for the differences between Asians and Caucasians lies with the alleles that affect the neurochemistry of the neural crest cells. Nature works in unpredictable and usually mysterious ways.

Asian and European Philosophies

These scattered pieces of evidence invite speculation on the reasons for the different philosophies favored by earlier generations of Asians and Europeans. Perhaps the most significant difference is that the first Greek philosophers, and later physical scientists, followed Democritus and assumed that permanent, indestructible atoms were the foundation of all matter. Buddhist scholars assumed that nothing was permanent. In addition, post-Reformation Protestant philosophy claimed that humans were inherently anxious and melancholic. The descriptions of human nature by Martin Luther and John Calvin emphasized the worry and guilt that were endemic to the human condition. Listen to Luther: "Should it not be enough for miserable sinners, eternally damned by original sin, to be oppressed by all sorts of calamity through the laws of the Ten Commandments? Must God add suffering to suffering through the Gospel and threaten us with His righteousness and His wrath through the Gospel, too?" John Calvin, who was chronically anxious, believed that humans could never escape the debilitating emotion of worry. One of Calvin's biographers remarked that his belief that freedom from anxiety was the most desirable of all states reflected a stoic view of beatitude that emanated from his profoundly melancholic mood. Unlike European literature from the eleventh to the eighteenth centuries, Japanese and Chinese literature rarely made conflicts of conscience over abstract religious or moral issues the central theme of a novel. There is no poem or novel in Asian literature comparable to Milton's *Paradise Lost* or Dante's *Divine Comedy* and no hero like Thomas More, who was willing to die for his religious beliefs. Shuichi Kato points out that Japanese novels during this era centered on maintaining harmonious social relationships and the pleasures of sex.

Buddhist philosophy, which was attractive to Asians, emphasized the attainment of serenity as life's goal. Each person approached this ideal state by ridding the self of desires because frustrated wishes were the primary cause of human unhappiness. Individuals could not attain tranquillity until they obliterated all conscious awareness of the world. This detachment of self from the world and people, which is required to gain Nirvana, is captured in the following story: "A monk was meditating under a tree when a former wife came and laid his child before him, saying, 'Here, monk, here is your little son, nourish me and nourish him.' The monk took no notice and sent her away. The Buddha, seeing this, said, 'He feels no pleasure when she comes, no sorrow when she goes, I call him a true Brahman released from passion.'" Contemporary American psychologists and psychiatrists, especially those friendly to attachment theory, would regard the monk as suffering from serious depression and in need of immediate therapy.

Sadness and regret, which accompany the failure to obtain a desired goal, have an experiential quality that differs from the anxiety or guilt that accompanies self-reproach or anticipated criticism from peers or from God. Put plainly, worry and sadness belong to distinctive emotional families. Moreover, the wish to eliminate high levels of affective arousal, whether pleasant or unpleasant, is linked to a more passive, rather than an active, attitude toward the world. I suspect that very few European philosophers would have celebrated the detached state of quiet passivity that the Chinese philosopher Lao-tzu praised almost 2,500 years ago:

Strength and power lie below, weakness and softness stand above
In all of the world, nothing is more pliant than water.
And yet it has no equal resiliency against that which is hard.
That which is weaker conquers that which is strong;
That which is soft conquers that which is hard . . .
There is nothing better than limitation.

Confucius had advocated the same approach to life five centuries earlier: "To remain unembittered even though one is unrecognized, is that not to be a noble man?"

Compare this celebration of a passive, unemotional acceptance of life's limitations with the contrasting view of Pierre Janet, the nineteenth-century French psychiatrist whose work was a foundation for Freud's ideas: "Sadness is always a sign of weakness and sometimes a habit of living weakly. The investigations with pathological psychology have shown us the evil of sadness and at the same time have evidenced a very important thing: the value of work and of joy."

Sophocles held the same opinion two thousand years earlier: "Sweetest of all things is this: the power each day to seize what one most wants."

Scholars commenting on the distinction between a philosophy that encourages the quiet acceptance of a life without desire or recrimination and one that demands an active coping with all obstacles in order to attain prized goals have usually emphasized only the role of culture and ecology. Most residents of ancient China, from about 500 BCE to the fifteenth century, lived in agricultural societies made up of small, ethnically homogeneous villages in which amicable relationships were mandatory. In addition, this large region experienced frequent natural catastrophes in the form of unpredictable floods, droughts, and earthquakes that would have provoked a passive posture toward a world that was uncontrollable. During the same era Europeans enjoyed a more benign climate and developed a larger commercial economy that required solitary individuals to take risks and to interact with different groups holding diverse values.

Nonetheless, I am tempted to suggest that the genomes of the two groups, through their influence on temperamental biases, made a small but real contribution to the differential attractiveness of each of these ideologies. If a large number of adults possessed a neurochemistry accompanied by high levels of body arousal that were interpreted as anxiety, guilt, or a desire for new pleasures, a philosophy advising them to be serene, free of desire, and detached from others would meet resistance because those states did not resemble the usual feeling tone they lived with each day.

As a result, the Asian view of Nirvana would appear to be both unreasonable and unattainable to most Europeans.

By contrast, a philosophy that accepted chronic anxiety, guilt, and frustrated wishes as definitive of the human condition would seem less valid to those whose consciousness was characterized by a typically lower level of arousal. The possibility of being free of the disturbing intrusiveness of strong, unpleasant feelings might seem a real possibility to this latter group. It is relevant that the traditional Chinese, along with other Asians, regarded the body as a vessel containing a limited amount of energy, called ch'i, that had to be preserved rather than expended. By contrast, Freud believed that the energy of the libido was to be invested in others and in activities that brought pleasure. Repression of libidinal energy produced neurotic symptoms, not serenity. The Chinese who use illicit drugs prefer opiates, which induce a feeling of relaxation. The Caucasians who abuse drugs prefer cocaine or amphetamines, which create increased arousal. Perhaps culture and genes came together, like the black and white threads of a seamless gray tapestry, to influence the philosophies that each of these groups adopted.

The Implication of Ethnic Differences

The profound effects of culture, social class, and social experiences on the course of individual development usually dominate the influences of genes. My earlier metaphor referring to the homogeneously gray cloth woven from the black threads of temperament and the white threads of experience also applies to the relation between the genomes of isolated populations and their cultures' practices. The genetic differences among world populations are small in an absolute sense, and alterations in the natural environment along with globalization of commerce and changing political structures can affect the observed outcomes of these genes.

More important, the genetic differences among reproductively isolated human groups have no political or legal implications. Women have higher basal metabolic rates and less muscle mass than men, but most democratic societies see no reason to use these features as a basis for awarding or restricting privileges to females. Unfortunately, many humans are tempted to evaluate any group difference as good or bad. Therefore, the possible existence of variation among ethnic groups in temperamental biases arouses strong emotion. When our understanding of the genetic and temperamental profiles of all human groups is more complete, which should occur during the next two centuries, we will learn that isolated populations possess special constellations of temperaments. But I suspect that the evidence will also indicate that each population possesses some biases that are adaptive in their society and some that are maladaptive. Hence, the account will be balanced. Suppose, for the sake of illustration, scientists discover that Caucasian females are at a slightly higher risk for depression than females with an African pedigree, but the African females are at slightly greater risk for developing diabetes. Or perhaps we will learn that Asians possess a temperamental profile that favors superior talent on spatial reasoning problems but also possess genes that make the possibility of suicide more probable. These examples imply that when all the evidence is in, we will appreciate that the alleles unique to each human group have both advantages and disadvantages.

There is no basis, either logical or empirical, for passing laws or implementing social practices that treat groups with distinctive genomes in a special way. Even the biologists who believe that human behavior should be viewed in a biological perspective do not insist that our moral evaluations or laws should accommodate only to scientific facts. They stop short of declaring that what is true in nature should be the only basis for deciding what human characteristics are good. Truth is a feature that applies to statements about the world, not to people. The adjectives "good" and "bad" apply to people and their actions.

Unfortunately, modern capitalist societies force many adults to be more competitive and aggressive than they would like, and they search for a rationale that might excuse excessive display of these qualities. When biologists declare that a fierce competitiveness that ignores the welfare of others is "natural," many citizens interpret that statement as meaning that this behavioral style is morally acceptable. Hence, each person can cover such actions with a veil of morality that makes the behavior not only necessary but also virtuous—like the kings or tribal chiefs in many ancient societies who asked astrologers or shamans to decide when to attack an enemy and when to plant spring crops.

A great deal of conflict might have been avoided if eighteenth-century Americans had not been keen on basing their ethics and laws on what was true in nature. During the century prior to the Civil War, many arguments for or against the morality of slavery hinged on whether Negroes were a member of the same species as whites. If yes, then Negroes had to be awarded freedom. If not, slave owners were justified in denying them liberty. Empirical facts were the basis for deciding what was an ethical issue. Why did eighteenth-century Americans look to science for authority? Why did they, and why do we, continue to regard scientific facts as the best defense of a moral proposition?

One reason is that scientific facts are presumably objective because they are derived from nature rather than human opinion. Therefore, they seem to be impartial, fair, and just. Moreover, science has gained the respect of the community through humanitarian advances, technical feats that magnify our sense of potency, and the prediction of a few future moments. As a result, science and a rational approach to experience have acquired a power that makes it easy for citizens to think that scientific knowledge is the best guide to morals and legislation.

The natural sciences confessed at the beginning of the last century, however, that their knowledge had no moral implications, because nature is value-free. Hence, citizens would have to look elsewhere for ethical guidance. As the nineteenth century came to a close, many European intellectuals were elaborating Kant's distinction between knowledge and values and assenting to Kierkegaard's plea to recognize the unbridgeable chasm between what is known and what is good. Ethics could never be found in reason, but only in each person's faith. But many in our society were not receptive to that declaration. Because neither the church nor philosophers were able to supply a persuasive rationale for morality in the twentieth century, scientists stepped forward to fill the breach, promising to solve the problems of ethical guidance by gathering objective information on questions with moral implications for the larger community. I am not sure, however, that the social or biological sciences can keep their promise.

Some anthropologists believe that studies of apes or non-modern cultures might reveal the basic nature of humanity and tell us how to construct an ethics that is consonant with nature's wishes rather than in opposition to them. It is unlikely, however, that studies of chimpanzees or other cultures can serve that function. One species of ape, called gibbons, are loyal to their mate and resemble prairie voles; gorillas, by contrast, do not bond to a single partner. Furthermore, bonobo chimpanzees have sex when they are upset, but a closely related strain of chimpanzees becomes aggressive when upset. It is not obvious, therefore, which species is the best model for humans—should we make love or war? Males, apes and humans, are sexually more promiscuous than females, but that scientific fact does not mean that we should change our laws regarding adultery.

Most Americans believe that the expression of anger is in accord with nature, and parents allow their children to display some aggression when frustrated or attacked and tell their children to defend themselves if coerced or bullied. Many also assume that if anger and hostility were always suppressed children might develop psychosomatic symptoms. However, Jean Briggs, who observed the Utku Eskimos of Hudson Bay, challenged the idea that suppression of hostility has unwanted consequences. Every display of anger or tantrums by an Utku child older than age two is followed by adult indifference; essentially the child receives the "silent treatment." Initially, the children are upset; however, after a year or two of this regimen tantrums vanish and aggression toward others is rare. Colitis, headaches, and other psychological symptoms that are supposed to result from the suppression of anger and aggression are also notably absent. Thus the answer to the question "Is it basic for humans to express anger or to suppress it?" is "Neither." The consequences of suppressing hostility always depend on the social context. It is maladaptive for individuals who live in an igloo nine months of the year to allow the expression of anger in any form, and this suppression does not lead to psychosomatic symptoms.

Each species, like the members of a culture, tries to adapt to its local conditions. Therefore, it is doubtful that any one species or culture can provide the "proper" model for human societies in the twenty-first century. If our ethics cannot find a foundation in scientific facts, where can we find a rationale for a moral code? One important source lies with the views of the majority, which, of course, change with time. Most Americans regard violence, dishonesty, intolerance, and coercion as morally indefensible, and a referendum on each would reflect that belief. Indeed, on election day many moral issues are placed on local ballots, suggesting the community's receptivity to using public sentiment as a guide to the solution of ethical dilemmas. When the Supreme Court recognized the difficulty of defining pornography objectively, the justices decided that local attitudes should determine the books and movies that violated local sensibility. The court legitimized the community's emotional reaction as a determinant of values.

The pragmatic spirit in America is one reason for some opposition to an ethically neutral attitude regarding the genetic differences among human populations. Americans are reluctant to celebrate knowledge that does not have some useful purpose, even though Congress voted millions of dollars to place telescopes in the sky in order to learn more about the earliest moments of our universe. This knowledge serves understanding and does not have obvious pragmatic implications. The products of science are one of the most powerful ways to illuminate many aspects of our world. The scientific conclusions that are constructed from the mysterious marriage of the concrete and the imagined evoke an emotional blend that combines clarity of comprehension with a feeling of awe or wonder for which English has no name. However, we still ask for more. Not satisfied with the gift of a more satisfying comprehension, we also demand that the fruits of all research be applied in some way, or at least help us decide what we should do when we have to choose one action over another. We must never forget, however, that scientific facts about brains, animals, or cultures, considered alone, can never be the basis of a moral premise. Facts can prune the tree of morality, but they can never be the seedbed.

6

Temperament and
Mental Illness

H istory's muse enjoys playing with the meanings of words, and
the events of the past two centuries have altered the meanings
of "mental illness" and its semantic relatives "mental disorder" and
"psychopathology." A majority of nineteenth-century American
and European physicians restricted the diagnosis of *mental illness* to
the small number of patients who had obviously deviant thoughts,
habits, or emotions that prevented them from meeting their responsibilities as students, spouses, parents, employees, or members of
the community. The relatively rare person who had hallucinations,
delusions of grandeur, or cycles of manic excitement followed by a
deep depression was viewed as a biological misfit who was qualitatively different from everyone else in the society. The ancient Greek
essayist Plutarch described a man who thought he was Alexander
the Great. Unfortunately, he was put to death because officials were
afraid his condition was a portent of the future.

Until recently, chronic unhappiness did not qualify as an illness as
long as a person appeared rational, socialized her children properly,

and carried out her work assignments reasonably well. Adults who drank too much, abused a spouse, lied regularly, worked in brothels, or engaged in criminal activity were judged amoral, and presumably harbored degenerate genes, but were not classified with those who believed they were Napoleon, heard the voice of their dead grandmother, or ran naked down the street yelling obscenities.

It is easy to understand the attractiveness of this narrow biological perspective on mental illness. Most nineteenth-century families lived in small communities in which a majority of parents treated their children similarly. Therefore, anyone who heard the voice of a dead ancestor, claimed to be Alexander the Great, or cycled between hurling unprovoked insults at friends and shuffling around the home all day in pajamas was both rare and puzzling, and it was reasonable to assume that a serious biological defect was responsible for their abnormal symptoms. Nineteenth-century neurologists would have agreed with the suggestion that these patients were born with an uncommon and debilitating temperamental bias.

Sigmund Freud challenged this view by introducing four new ideas as the new century began. First, he rejected the strict biological determinism of his contemporaries and inserted the vague, psychobiological concept of anxiety between the presumed compromise in brain function and the disturbing emotions and behaviors. This suggestion implied that the patient's psychological state was a critical phase in a cascade that began in the brain and ended in a mental illness. Second, the source of anxiety was a buildup of energy caused by repression of ideas related to sexuality. But the energy linked to these ideas would be weakened if they were made conscious. Third, Freud insisted that the patient's early experiences, and especially those within the family, were the most important origins of the anxiety that was the critical cause of the symptoms. Finally, Freud implied that anyone exposed to childhood events that created high levels of anxiety could acquire the symptoms of mental illness. This bold suggestion meant that everyone was potentially at risk, not just the small number of people with faulty genes. Thus, a bout of intense worry or sadness at least once in a lifetime, which is experienced by more than 25 percent of adults living in contemporary developed societies, has become a sign of a mental illness.

Freud's radical proposals were greeted with applause by politically liberal social scientists and the educated Americans who were eager to assimilate the poor, often illiterate European immigrants settling in large numbers in our cities. These citizens were troubled by the attempts of many eminent Americans to pressure Congress to pass laws requiring sterilization of the mentally ill or retarded and restricting future immigration. American social scientists were reluctant to attribute the academic failures and delinquent acts of the children of these immigrants to degenerate genes or a damaged brain. They wanted to prove that the causes of these undesirable characteristics were environmental and, therefore, potentially able to be remedied.

At the center of Freud's explanation of mental symptoms was the implication that parental interactions with the child, in the form of love and a gentle discipline that did not create excessive guilt, provided protection against future pathology. If parents were too harsh, rejecting, or negligent, they would establish the foundation for later symptoms. Freud did not waffle in his classic 1936 monograph, *The Problem of Anxiety*, when he stated that the fearful reactions infants show to the dark, to being alone, or to a stranger were examples of the same fundamental emotion; namely, "feeling the loss of the loved (longed for) person," which in most instances was the mother. This bold, but unverified, idea was treated as a profound insight. Only fifty years ago a majority of American and European psychiatrists and psychologists were certain that an aloof, insensitive mother could create the seriously debilitating symptoms that define childhood autism. I know no clinician or scientist who would defend that idea today.

The initial popularity of Freud's account of mental illness, especially in America and England, profited from a number of novel historical conditions that emerged during the last decade of the nineteenth century and the first two decades of the twentieth. The first cars, buses, planes, telephones, electric lights, and cinemas required new forms of energy that obeyed physical laws. These machines generated an excitement blended with apprehension because cars and planes seemed to pose dangers. Second, the growth of cities, due to expanded sources of employment, motivated many young women to leave their rural homes and migrate to urban areas, where they interacted with men looking for sexual partners. The recent introduction of inexpensive condoms allowed many of these unmarried women to consider sexual affairs without the fear of pregnancy, and sexual images, many of them pornographic, were penetrating the ordinary literature as well as the art of European culture. Despite sexuality's fuller access to consciousness, these ideas and feelings still evoked a blend of anxiety, shame, and guilt. Third, all forms of traditional authority, along with their assumptions, were being challenged, including the status of women and their demand for an education, the right to vote, and sexual pleasures equivalent to those of men. This celebration of personal liberty and self-actualization, which was stronger in America and England than in the societies of Continental Europe, made Freud's message more attractive to those living in these two Protestant countries. Finally, Freud was probably influenced by the hypocrisy of Viennese society. This mood had become so transparent that social commentators argued that the surface of a society presented a false picture and its true nature lay hidden beneath the public actions and casual conversations. This idea was buttressed by the recent invention of the X-ray, which provided a concrete example of the psychoanalytic premise that the causes of people's essential character resided in their unconscious rather than in their conscious understandings or explanations to others.

When humans are aroused by vague feelings with puzzling origins, they search for a reasonable interpretation that is congruent with the views of respected authority. Because the physicists' concept of energy enjoyed high respect, Freud's intuition that the energy associated with repressed psychological ideas obeyed similar laws made his theory attractive, even though there was absolutely no support for this bold premise. Freud invented a creative metaphor when he implied that the weakening of a repressed desire through remembering and confessing it to another rested on a process that resembled the loss of energy in a closed vessel of hot water that had been exposed to the open air. Second, the desires for money, fame, status, and beautiful children were old, familiar wishes. The wish to be free of traditional constraints on strong desires, especially the motive to have frequent sex with more people, was a novel idea, and as a result, thoughts about sex became a hub around which the mind circled continually, not unlike the rough spot on a tooth to which the tongue reflexively returns. Therefore, Freud's suggestion that the repression of sexual desire was the primary cause of the anxiety that produced unwanted symptoms seemed correct to those who accepted the energy metaphor and were threatened by the new, dehumanizing technologies, the challenge to traditional authority, and the ascendance of women. Put plainly, sexual frustration was nominated as the sole origin of a blend of excitement and uncertainty that was actually due to a host of different historical conditions. If Freud had been able to read the diary of a thirteenth-century merchant traveling through Arabia, he would have realized the flaw in his ideas. The residents of this region had minimal shame or guilt over sexuality but were extremely violent and vulnerable to bouts of anxiety and depression.

A century later, a new collection of novelties—cell phones, the Internet, DVDs, fax machines—allowed large numbers of professionals to work and play in solitude. At the same time, new business arrangements required many workers to move to a different city every few years and raise their families in neighborhoods of strangers. It is not surprising that John Cacioppo, an eminent University of Chicago psychologist, and William Patrick, a science editor, wrote a book a few years ago claiming that the lack of close, trusting relationships with others, not restrained sexuality, was an important cause of anxiety and melancholia.

I suspect that the novelties of 2110, which cannot be anticipated, will generate yet another explanation for the bouts of worry, guilt, shame, anger, and sadness that, like hunger and bruised knees, are permanent features of the human condition. Neither repression of sexuality nor the absence of friends, when defined objectively, is the origin of anxiety or depression across historical eras and cultures. Rather, the main causes of these uncomfortable emotions are the conceptions of the psychological resources and mental states that individuals believe they ought to command or those that violate their understanding of what is morally right. An unmarried keeper of a lighthouse who liked his job and did not interpret his social isolation as implying that he was inadequate, less worthy, or less deserving of grace would not develop intense anxiety or depression. The reason an anxiety-ridden sexuality in 1900 and a lack of close relationships in 2010 generate unwanted feelings is that many interpret both states as inconsistent with what they have been led to believe are the qualities that a virtuous, and well-adjusted person is supposed to possess. Many contemporary twenty-five-year-old American women have been persuaded that they should experience orgasm during every sexual intimacy, and some seek professional help if they cannot attain this state regularly. Most eighteenth-century American women would not have decided that they had a psychological impairment requiring therapy if they did not have an orgasm every time they made love. Freud failed to recognize that the villain was not repressed sexual desire but a private interpretation of that condition implying that the self was less healthy, less in tune with nature's intention, and, therefore, a less worthy person.

It is relevant that a number of Freud's first disciples and advocates, including Karen Horney, Melanie Klein, and Helene Deutsch, were well-educated European women who were the vanguard of the movement that burgeoned sixty years later demanding more freedom for women from male domination. America's eroticization of each person's freedom to pursue personal interests lent authority to Freud's argument that individuals would move toward greater health and vitality if they liberated the desires imprisoned in their unconscious. A popular psychology textbook of 1930 declared, without evidence, that the primary goal of human development was the emancipation of children from the restrictions their families imposed on them. Thus, the receptivity to Freud's statement that psychoanalysis "sets a neurotic free from the chains of his sexuality" benefited from the semantic link between the motto on the New Hampshire license plate, "Live free or die," and the networks of ideas and feelings surrounding sexual gratification that lay shackled in the dark dungeon of the unconscious. Freud was acutely aware of his minority status as a Jew in anti-Semitic Austrian society and must have hoped that he could be free of the anxiety and vigilant posture that accompanied his awareness of the prejudice directed at all who shared his ethnicity and religion.

Finally, Freudian ideas implied that everyone, potentially, could rid themselves of the uncomfortable state of anxiety, either by entering into psychoanalysis or by yielding to their wishes for more pleasure. The notion that humans could, and should, be free of all anxiety, as the Salk vaccine eliminated polio, is one of the distinguishing illusions in Western thought. Unfortunately, episodes of anxiety can never be eliminated from the psyche because uncertainty over future threats is as inherent in the human condition as a painful muscle strain.

Psychoanalytic ideas were less popular in Continental Europe than in America during Freud's lifetime because Europeans strove for a healthier balance between maintaining the harmony of the community and gratifying the self's wishes. Europeans were willing to accept some restrictions on their personal freedom if those restraints strengthened their community. Paris and Florence were vibrant cities long before New York and Chicago had paved streets. Furthermore, many European countries had suffered from centuries of wars initiated by men with an exaggerated sense of self who failed to suppress their strong wish for power. Hence, the average European was a bit more skeptical of Freud's claim that the celebration of an unfettered ego rebelling against the mores of society was a wise philosophy.

The Return to Biology

The Freudian revolution, which was helped by the American behaviorists' emphasis on the role of experience, enjoyed considerable ideological dominance for almost sixty years. Most American commentators on development in the 1920s announced confidently that all mental illness could be traced to improper parental treatment. However, this narrative changed in the 1970s, for two reasons.

First, faith in psychoanalytic theory eroded because the prevalence of anxiety and depression did not decrease, despite the lifting of repression on sexuality and the failure to validate Freud's predictions of the effects of certain early experiences, such as abrupt weaning or harsh toilet training. Freud made a serious error when he inserted two personal ethical premises into his theory—namely, that sexual restraint was always unhealthy and that societies interfered with the optimal psychological development of their citizens. Darwin, by contrast, understood that there are no moral values in nature; herons are not superior to hens.

The second cause of the new point of view was that neuroscientists and molecular biologists, armed with powerful new techniques that could measure brain states and genes, placed biology, once again, in the villainous role of the cause of mental illness. The return to a strong form of biological influence found an especially receptive audience among younger scientists. The erosion in the quality of instruction in urban schools, due partly to the abandonment of teaching as a career by well-educated, dedicated women who could become lawyers, doctors, business executives, or scientists, led to a rise in the proportion of youth who were unable to read, write, or solve arithmetic problems. A generation earlier, many Americans would have blamed the families of the failing children for not encouraging greater perseverance in the classroom. But after the civil rights movement of the 1960s, it became politically incorrect to blame poor African American or Hispanic families for the high rates of academic failure among their children. One alternative was to attribute the inadequate achievement to the child's biology. Once this happened, the frequency of diagnoses of learning disability, dyslexia, and attention-deficit/hyperactivity disorder soared.

At the same time, the availability of drugs that promised to alleviate anxiety, depression, and hyperactivity persuaded many psychiatrists to prescribe medicines rather than psychotherapy for a troubled adult or a tutor for a failing child. This heavy reliance on pills was helped by the fact that medical insurance companies were perfectly willing to pay for pills, but less willing to reimburse doctors for six months of psychotherapy or to compensate families for payments to a college student helping a child learn to read. If the chemicals in a pill reduced the seriousness of a symptom, it seemed reasonable to conclude that a chemical must also be the cause. This logic won the day, even though physicians knew that shoveling too much snow was the reason for the pain of a muscle strain that was reduced by several capsules of Advil. Unfortunately, the mechanisms that explain a cure are rarely the same as those that cause the symptom.

Finally, Americans and Europeans remained attracted to the ancient Greek intuition, supported by most natural scientists in succeeding centuries, that material things—atoms, molecules, and neurons—were the foundation of all psychological phenomena. Thoughts, wishes, and feelings, which were not material things, must be derivative processes of secondary significance that could be explained by a material brain. All these factors came together, like a perfect storm, to catapult biological mechanisms into the position of the alpha cause of most mental illnesses and to return the ancient notion of temperament to its earlier prominence, with brain chemicals replacing blood, phlegm, and yellow and black bile as the critical cause of symptoms.

Mismatch between Temperament and Psychiatric Categories

A more profound appreciation of the temperamental contribution to psychiatric illnesses has evaded us because psychiatrists routinely categorize mental illnesses from the patients' verbal descriptions of their symptoms. These statements ignore the causal power of temperaments as well as the patient's past history and current life circumstances. Most patients fail to mention some of these features because the information is unavailable to consciousness. This indifference to the origins of a symptom is unfortunate, because every contemporary category in the psychiatrist's diagnostic manual (called the *Diagnostic and Statistical Manual of Mental Disorders*, or *DSM*) has more than one pattern of causal conditions. That is, each mental illness is the product of more than one combination of temperamental biases and life histories. Thus it is difficult to detect the effect of a particular temperamental bias on any one of the psychiatric categories. The problem with relying only on reported symptoms is that there are far fewer symptoms than there are combinations of molecules, brain circuits, and experience.

Paul McHugh, formerly a director of the department of psychiatry at the Johns Hopkins University School of Medicine, explained in the book *Try to Remember* why the current *DSM* psychiatric categories became popular. In the 1970s, psychiatrists recognized that they needed a classification system that would allow a majority of psychiatrists to agree on who was paranoid, depressed, or anxious. In the past, doctors had not been able to agree on a diagnosis because they used idiosyncratic inferences about the patient's unconscious conflicts based on the patient's history. Agreement would improve if the illness categories were defined only by presenting symptoms. The symptoms' presumed origins in biology or the patient's history were to be ignored. The professionals who wrote the manual also assumed that if a committee of experienced psychiatrists believed that a particular illness category existed, it must be a real phenomenon. In a few instances, that premise may be unjustified. For example, the manual describes a mental illness called "multiple personality disorder," which McHugh believes does not exist.

Most psychiatrists also ignore the different qualities of emotions for which English has only one word. Humans are vulnerable to different qualities of sadness and depression following rejection by a lover, chronic poverty, loss of a job, the inability to complete a project, the unexpected death of an infant, or betrayal by a close friend or spouse. A majority of psychiatrists ignore these differences and place all individuals who report being chronically sad and apathetic into a category called "depressive disorder." For all of these reasons, it is impossible to determine the influence of any one temperamental bias on these heterogeneous psychiatric categories as long as psychiatrists ignore the origins of a symptom profile. Biologists would not have discovered some of the genes that render a woman vulnerable to a form of breast cancer if they had pooled all adults with a cancer of any organ into one omnibus category.

A New Classification

The need for a new set of categories that acknowledges the joint influence of temperament and past history motivated McHugh to assign each of the mental illnesses to one of four heterogeneous families defined by unique combinations of symptoms and causes. This strategy is analogous to assigning each physical disease to one of four major families defined by its origin: viral or bacterial infections, cancerous growths, circulatory problems, or metabolic errors. Each of these families contains different illnesses, but those in the same family share a few features unique to that family.

McHugh's classifications rest upon three critical assumptions. First, each of the four families contains patients with different combinations of biological vulnerabilities and past histories. Second, anxiety or depression can be present in patients belonging to any of the families. Third, a person can develop some symptoms as the result of a life history of stress or current challenges without possessing a special temperamental vulnerability.

I add four ideas to McHugh's trio of reasonable assumptions. First, a precipitating event is often necessary to transform a temperamental vulnerability into the symptoms of a mental illness. Some adolescents who are vulnerable to becoming anxious or depressed develop these symptoms only if they encounter a new set of challenges—for example, leaving home to attend a college many miles away. Had they attended a college close to home, the serious symptoms might not have appeared at that time. Young American girls are vulnerable to a bout of depression if they develop breasts much earlier than their peers, because they feel different from other girls and have to cope with sexual advances from boys. Boys are prone to a depressed mood if their physical development is delayed, because being shorter and less muscular than their friends renders them vulnerable to teasing and victimization by bullies.

Second, the patient's interpretations of events, not the events that a camera would record, are the primary cause of many, but not all, symptoms. If the victims of a crime, earthquake, flood, or tsunami interpret the disaster as implying either that they are partially responsible for their distress or have become vulnerable to further catastrophes, they are more likely to develop the symptoms of post-traumatic stress disorder. Those who regard the disaster as a purely chance event with no implications for their virtue or future safety are protected from these symptoms. Only some rape victims decide they are partially to blame for the attack; only some depressed patients conclude that their unhappiness is a punishment for past ethical violations. When people are convinced that they made a willful contribution to their condition, a corrosive guilt is added to their existing emotional state. By contrast, if individuals believe that the cause of their distress was the actions of others, anger becomes the dominant emotion. Chronically poor Americans feel anger toward many in their society; affluent adults who lost their wealth due to poor investment decisions are prone to guilt.

A person's cultural background often colors the individual's interpretation of an event or psychological state. Depressed or anxious women living in the towns or villages of seventeenth-century Germany who had yielded to the sexual advances of a stranger when younger were tempted years later to explain their current distress by saying that the seducing stranger had been the devil and therefore they must be a witch. Some contemporary German women with the same symptoms accept their therapists' suggestion that their father's sexual abuse of them when they were children, which they have repressed, is the cause of their current distress.

Many well-educated, economically secure women from New York who feel apathetic decide to exercise and reduce their intake of carbohydrates. When working-class, immigrant women from south Asia who live in the same city have similar feelings, they eat more carbohydrates, go to bed, or visit a nearby mosque to renew their religious commitment. A tribe of Salteaux Indians living near Lake Winnipeg in Canada is not afraid of the many bears in the region, even though some hunters have been injured by bears, but they become very anxious if a bear enters the area where families live, because they interpret that intrusion as meaning that someone in the village has been bewitched.

Less than a century ago many Americans believed that a child who masturbated was at risk of becoming "crazy." Freud believed that a man who engaged in intercourse but did not ejaculate, or practiced coitus interruptus, was at risk for serious mental symptoms. Contemporary Americans over age fifty who are barraged with ads for Viagra are susceptible to deciding that the absence of regular sexual gratification is a threat to their health. The main point is that all humans, no matter how sophisticated, are vulnerable to worry if they interpret a state of affairs that poses no objective threat as a sign of danger.

The unfamiliarity or unexpectedness of a stressful condition that provokes anxiety or depression is a third factor affecting the intensity of the emotions surrounding the symptom. A college senior who always obtained high scores on examinations, from the first grade through the junior year, is apt to become unusually upset upon receiving a first failing grade. An investor who has never lost a great deal of money will be prone to anxiety and/or guilt following a large loss. The members of upper-middle-class Jewish families living in Austria and Germany who suddenly lost their status and wealth in 1938 when Hitler assumed power became vulnerable to nightmares, bouts of depression, or chronic anxiety that in some cases lasted a lifetime, even if they escaped Nazi concentration camps. The quality of these emotional reactions to the same events is different in those who occasionally fail examinations, never had a great deal of money, or have always occupied the less-advantaged social ranks in a society.

Finally, the patients' belief that they can do something to alleviate their symptoms is relevant. The intensity of anxiety or depression is far more distressing if patients conclude that they are helpless. All societies provide their members with ritual actions that are supposed to reduce the level of worry over one's health and wealth. Despite several excellent studies indicating that adults who eat a balanced diet do not profit from taking vitamin or herbal supplements, it is hard to dissuade them from this morning ritual because humans demand that there is something they can do to mute uncertainty over their health. Those who believe there is no action they can implement to alleviate their worry, shame, or guilt are susceptible to a profound melancholy.

McHugh's Four Families

I now describe four symptom families that have their origin in (1) serious brain pathology, (2) temperamental biases for anxiety or depression, (3) temperamental biases that make it difficult to regulate impulsive behavior, or (4) life circumstances.

Family 1

The first family of psychological disorders is defined by serious deficits in attention, memory, reasoning, language, or states of consciousness. These symptoms are more common in males, have the lowest prevalence of the four categories, and their frequency has changed the least over the past century. The symptoms of this family are usually the result of inherited abnormalities in brain anatomy or chemistry, but can be the product of a brain infection or, in some cases, compromises in brain function that accompany aging. The patients in this family are usually diagnosed as schizophrenic, bipolar, or autistic, and examination of their brains with magnetic scanners often detects one or more abnormalities.

However, the symptoms that define each of these diagnoses have more than one set of causes, and therefore none is a unitary disease with one origin. Moreover, the course of the illness can be influenced by the patient's gender and social class. For example, researchers who studied schizophrenic Israeli males found that those with more education and, by inference, were from more-advantaged backgrounds had a better prognosis than male patients who were economically disadvantaged.

Children are diagnosed with autism if they have serious impairments in language and social skills, and display inappropriate emotions and stereotyped motor acts, such as pulling their hair, rocking, or head banging. These symptoms, alone or in combination, can be the product of a large but still unknown number of distinct biological conditions, including alterations in genes or chromosomes, maternal illness during pregnancy, early postnatal infection, or a rare immune reaction in infancy. When I was a graduate student in the 1950s, most of these children were assigned the amorphous label "brain damaged." The word "damaged," for which "defective" is a close semantic associate, has stigmatic connotations that are missing from the less familiar term "autistic," for which "artistic" is a possible association.

Because the category "autistic" contains many distinct forms of mental illness, the popular practice of grouping all autistic individuals into a category called "the autistic spectrum" is a serious error. The same may be true for the diagnosis of schizophrenia. The number of diagnoses of autism rose by an extraordinary 600 percent in California between 1990 and 2003 because physicians were awarding this label to any child who showed signs of serious language delay, inappropriate social behavior, or stereotyped motor acts. The practice of pooling diseases with diverse causes into one diagnostic group will delay discovery of the unique biological characteristics and best therapy for each disease. No physician would group all patients complaining of headaches into a category called "the headache spectrum," because they know that headaches can be the result of a diverse set of qualitatively different conditions, each requiring a different treatment. Furthermore, because autistic patients are qualitatively different from normal children, it is not obvious that we will learn much by comparing the scores of these children on tests of single cognitive abilities with the scores of normal children. This strategy assumes that the group called autistic and all healthy children vary only quantitatively in memory or language abilities. If the organizations of memory and language skills are qualitatively different in children with autism, these studies have questionable value. No biologist would measure the difference between polio patients and healthy people by the time required by each to run a mile.

Family 2

McHugh's second family is characterized by reports of chronic or intense episodes of anxiety or depression due to various combinations of temperamental biases and life histories. The patients in this large family have qualitatively different symptom patterns, with names like phobic disorder, post-traumatic stress disorder, panic disorder, general anxiety disorder, obsessive-compulsive disorder, anorexia, and depression. Each of these seven categories contains illnesses with different origins, age of onset, and degree of heritability. Unlike the symptoms of family 1, those of family 2 are more common in females than males and are more often the result of an imbalance in brain chemistry than a serious anatomical abnormality. Moreover, many individuals in this family are able to meet most of their major responsibilities as parents, employees, or citizens despite their intense private distress. A few even achieve eminence in their society. John Calvin, the sixteenth-century Protestant reformer, Virginia Woolf and T. S. Eliot, twentieth-century writers, and Rita Levi-Montalcini, a Nobel laureate in biology, are examples of individuals who suffered at some time in their lives from intense bouts of anxiety or depression that may have contributed to their creative products. A critical biological feature of many patients in this family is abnormally high excitability in a set of connected brain structures, which include the amygdala and the anterior cingulate cortex. The profiles of excitability are the partial product of a large number of genes that affect the overall activity of serotonin, dopamine, norepinephrine, and the molecules that regulate the duration of their activity (figure 6). Therefore, a given level of excitability in any one of these structures could result from a variety of conditions. Individuals with high levels of excitability in these brain sites are vulnerable to exaggerated reactions to novel experiences or to situations in which they have to select the best action from several alternatives. As I noted earlier, an unfamiliar event provokes "event uncertainty;" the need to choose one course of action from a set of alternatives evokes "response uncertainty." Each state is associated with different symptoms.

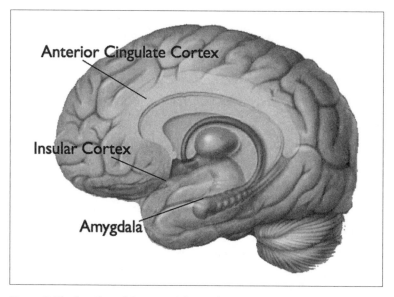

Figure 6. The location of the amygdala, insular cortex, and anterior cingulate cortex in the human brain.

Phobias

The defining symptoms in this category are consistent avoidance of particular objects or situations, accompanied by an uncomfortable feeling of anxiety. However, the person's temperament and past experience influence the specific object or situation that is avoided. Adults who say they are afraid of small insects, such as spiders and cockroaches, for example, are usually worried about being contaminated rather than about being harmed physically. This is not the reason why some patients have phobias about large dogs, tall buildings, or closed spaces.

Many patients who say they are afraid of blood or an injection possess a biology that is rare among most phobic patients; they have a very low systolic blood pressure, which renders them vulnerable to fainting when they see blood. By contrast, many patients with a fear of heights have a compromise in the inner ear, which is responsible for a sense of balance, and experience uncomfortable feelings when they look down from a high cliff or a tall building.

Perhaps the largest number of phobic patients avoid strangers and unfamiliar social situations, called social phobia or social anxiety disorder. Some have a vulnerability to facial flushing when they think they are being evaluated. The majority are unsure of how to behave with people they do not know, an example of response uncertainty. These individuals are not afraid of being harmed, contaminated, or fainting, but they worry that they will feel humiliated or embarrassed in the presence of others because of their appearance, language, absence of spontaneity, or lack of sophistication. Japanese adults with social phobia say that they avoid strangers because they do not want to disturb others with their awkward behavior. Americans with social phobia are more concerned with how they feel rather than with the feelings of others.

Social anxiety disorder includes two categories of patients. One type develops their symptoms before adolescence; the other group usually becomes anxious after the second or third decade. These two groups probably have distinctive temperaments. Among the early-onset group, the high-reactive infants described in chapter 2 are at the greatest risk for developing social phobia as adults. These individuals are tense when they meet strangers, hate to be part of a large crowd, and prefer solitary hobbies and vocations. Those who are lucky enough to find an adaptive niche that protects them from continuous encounters with unfamiliar people and situations often make a moderately successful adjustment and do not develop phobic symptoms requiring professional help. I noted that T. S. Eliot was an example of a person who obtained dignity, fame, and financial security despite a temperamental vulnerability for social anxiety.

PTSD

The category called post-traumatic stress disorder is defined by symptoms of intense anxiety, obsessive rumination, nightmares, or a severe numbing of emotion following an unexpected and statistically improbable trauma, especially the violence of war, rape, earthquake, flood, or a serious automobile accident. This disorder illustrates the importance of the patient's temperament, life circumstances, and the subjective interpretation imposed on a threatening experience. For example, although PTSD is more prevalent among women than men in most cultures, black males with a Caribbean pedigree living in America are an exception to this rule. These men are more likely than women of Caribbean descent to develop PTSD because they are more often involved in violent fights with peers.

Only a minority of children or adults exposed to a trauma develop the symptoms of PTSD because they possess a temperamental bias. For example, only ten of forty schoolchildren who were kidnapped and terrorized for more than two days developed the debilitating symptoms. Similarly, only one-third of young children attending a Los Angeles elementary school who witnessed a sniper kill one child and injure eighteen was seriously anxious one month later. An equal proportion were free of any disabling emotion. Moreover, the children who remained anxious had been timid and avoidant prior to the violence, implying that they possessed a temperamental bias that made them susceptible to the symptoms of PTSD. The small number of children who remained anxious seven months after Hurricane Andrew struck the region in which they lived had also been classified as extremely fearful many months before the hurricane arrived.

Some who develop PTSD interpret the traumatic event as implying that they have become especially vulnerable to life's dangers or feel guilty because they witnessed or participated in an amoral act. The latter occurred among soldiers who watched the torture of prisoners or the senseless killing of innocent civilians and could not rationalize the necessity for these horrific events. Prisoners who were tortured because of their political beliefs were protected from PTSD because they could explain why a regime victimized them. Ordinary criminals subjected to the same torture are denied this protection.

The victims of a catastrophe who regard the event as a rare, chance event over which they had no control are also protected from intense distress. Thirty years ago, a group of Iranians held a large number of Americans hostage for more than a year in a building in Tehran. The Americans were released soon after Ronald Reagan was inaugurated as president and were flown to an air force base in Germany, where they were examined by a team of psychiatrists and psychologists. Although all the hostages had experienced the same serious threat to their lives, some were relatively calm and reported that they had been certain that they would eventually be rescued unharmed. Those with the classic symptoms of PTSD were continually frightened because they were sure they would be killed. It is likely that the different temperaments and life histories of these two groups created these two distinct reactions to the same threat.

The intensity of a woman's emotional reaction to being raped is influenced by whether she believes she made a willful contribution to her victimization. An adolescent girl who was raped while walking home from a party at 2 a.m. will feel guilty and, therefore, more distressed if she realizes she could have walked home with a friend, taken a taxi, or left the party early. Kathryn Flynn, a California psychologist, interviewed eighteen women who had been sexually abused by clergy in the church they attended. These women suffered from nightmares, chronic jitteriness, an inability to stop thinking about the sexual encounters, or a shutting out of the experience.

One woman reported, "It was like being in hell, you know ... that's all I could think of. ... I was obsessed with this thing. ... I'm continually spinning my wheels about this thing ... it took over" Another woman denied the events: "I tend to block a lot of what happened out, so I don't recall everything. ... I had no idea ... if this really happened like this, or if I had had a nightmare. ... I had gotten to the point where I had actually confused myself about what had really happened."

Confusion over what is real and what is imagined is more common among children. My wife and I had returned from a trip to the Cincinnati zoo with our 2½-year-old daughter, who said she wanted to remain in the car. I put the car in gear (in 1957 cars had the gearshift on the wheel), and we went into the house. Several minutes later I heard a loud crash. I ran outside, saw no car, and raced to the edge of the lawn, where there was a one hundred-foot drop to the ground below. When I saw the crushed car at the bottom of this cliff, I scampered down and found that our daughter had been thrown into the backseat but appeared unharmed. The doctor who examined her forty minutes later declared that no bone had been broken, no concussion had occurred, and she seemed to be unaffected by the trauma.

Because I was still loyal to some Freudian ideas in 1957, I thought it wise to avoid any mention of the incident in order to prevent the development of a phobia of cars. And for the next twenty-three years neither my wife nor I mentioned this accident. But one December morning, when she was visiting for the Christmas holiday, I happened to ask her about her earliest memories, even though I was not thinking about the accident. She told me that for the past twenty-three years she had thought about the event on many occasions, but did not know if it had actually happened or if she had imagined it, and she chastised me for refusing to discuss the trauma. I experienced the nightmares characteristic of PTSD for several months after the incident, because I blamed myself for allowing my daughter to remain alone in the car.

Panic disorder

Adults with panic disorder suffer from a unique temperamental bias characterized by unusual sensitivity to bodily changes and unexpected surges of autonomic activity that are accompanied by a sharp increase in heart rate, difficulty breathing, or excessive perspiration. These unexpected sensations, believed to be due partly to a hyper-excitable insula, evoke uncertainty, and the individuals try to understand the reason for the surprising change in feeling. If they decide these feelings are signs of danger—for example, "I'm going crazy" or "I must be having a heart attack"—they become extremely distressed. If the attacks persist, some patients become afraid of leaving the security of their home because they worry that an autonomic surge might occur when they are driving on a highway. The combination of unexpected surges of bodily arousal and a catastrophic interpretation defines panic disorder. If individuals decide that the autonomic surges pose no danger, the extreme levels of anxiety are aborted and they are not diagnosed with panic disorder, even though they continue to live with a special sensitivity to bodily changes and occasional autonomic surges.

Anorexia

Patients suffering from anorexia who decide to stop eating for months or years, more often females, provide another example of how combinations of a temperamental bias and life circumstances can create serious symptoms. There are several different reasons why an adolescent or young adult woman would decide to restrict her intake of food. American society promotes the idea that being thin is a salient requirement for females who want to be physically attractive. Hence, many girls wishing to be more attractive develop anorexia after months on a starvation diet. A desire to feel virtuous by denying the self all sensory pleasures, or a wish to remain sexually immature by slowing the growth of breasts and hips in order to avoid being treated as a young adult with sexual interests, can also motivate the first phase of a cascade that ends in anorexia. The latter dynamic is common among young Japanese anorexic women, because Japanese girls are overprotected by their families and are anxious about assuming adult responsibilities.

A fourth basis for this symptom is a wish to reassure the self that it is still in control. A small proportion of adults possess a temperamental vulnerability to salient feelings of uncertainty when they cannot predict or prepare for the events of each day. This state is common among high-reactives. When local circumstances prevent these individuals from the tight management of their lives, this temperamental bias is transformed into anxiety and the symptoms of anorexia can begin. The belief that one is no longer able to anticipate what will happen in the next few hours or days motivates some young women to find an action that will reassure the self that it is still in charge of the day's events. One way to achieve this reassurance is to stop eating.

Laura Moisin, who had been anorexic, described this dynamic in a compelling memoir called *Kid Rex*. Laura was born with a temperament that rendered her vulnerable to uncertainty when she felt she could not control her immediate future. She was able to maintain certainty as a high school student in Newton, Massachusetts, for she studied diligently, received excellent grades, and lived in a protected family environment. Her anorexia began after she matriculated at New York University and lived in an apartment with several others in New York's Chinatown. The chaotic unpredictability of the setting was threatening and, in an attempt to seize some measure of control, she decided to stop eating, an act accompanied by the thought "I was strong enough to need no food." After trying several different therapists, she found one who helped her return to a normal life. I suspect that her anorexia might not have developed if she had attended a small college in a rural area. It is not uncommon for adolescents with a good adjustment in a protected atmosphere in a small town to develop serious mental symptoms during their first year away from home on a large college campus if they have the temperamental bias of a high-reactive infant.

The long-term consequences of an episode of anorexia during adolescence are not well understood. A team of Swedish scientists has provided us with some initial information by studying fifty-one anorexic adolescents (mainly girls and constituting 1 percent of the girls in the city of Goteborg) over an interval of eighteen years. Although half of this group of adults were no longer anorexic, about 50 percent of the "recovered" group developed other symptoms, especially an anxiety or depressive disorder. The half who not only recovered from anorexia but also appeared to be free of serious psychiatric illness as adults had acquired their anorexia later in adolescence and had not shown perfectionist rituals or compulsions during childhood. These facts imply that only some who develop anorexia have a temperamental bias for this disorder.

Obsessive-compulsive disorder
Patients are diagnosed with obsessive-compulsive disorder (OCD) if they develop any one of a variety of symptoms that include (1) obsessive thoughts they cannot suppress, usually about sex, religious blasphemy, or harming others, (2) a compulsion to hoard food, string, or old paper, (3) an urge to wash their hands every hour or two, or (4) repeated checking of a stove to see that it is turned

off or the back door to make sure it is locked. A small proportion of patients with one or more of these symptoms also have motor tics, such as frequent blinking, scratching a part of the body, or biting the bottom lip, which occur without conscious awareness.

OCD symptoms can also be the product of different temperamental biases and life histories. The patients who develop these symptoms during childhood are more often boys, whereas more adult patients are women. A small proportion of OCD patients who also have motor tics had an earlier streptococcus infection that damaged a part of the brain that participates in the circuit that mediates the tic. Only about half of adult OCD patients had symptoms as children, and only half of children with OCD continue to suffer from these symptoms as adults. Men and women possess different combinations of complaints. Female patients tend to combine a compulsion to clean with depressed moods and panic disorder. Male OCD patients more often combine obsessive thoughts with tics.

The content of the obsessive thoughts varies with the culture. Muslim men are bothered by intrusive thoughts with a religious content; Brazilian men obsess over aggression; Mexican men, over sexuality. The evidence, still incomplete, implies that a large number of OCD patients have an abnormally high level of excitability in a circuit that includes the underside of the prefrontal cortex (the orbitofrontal cortex), the anterior cingulate cortex (which contributes to the inhibition of unwanted responses), and a structure beneath the cortex (caudate nucleus) that mediates motor actions. The high level of excitability in the loop that connects these three sites implies some compromise in the brain processes that are supposed to maintain a balance between excitability and inhibition.

Depression

A diagnosis of depression is given to patients who report either a chronically sad, melancholic mood or a pervasive inability to extract pleasure from daily experience. Most report both states, although each state can be the result of different mechanisms. One of every eight people will have at least one serious bout of depression during their lifetime, and this mood will occur more often among females than among males (12 vs. 7 percent among Americans). Some depressed patients have secondary symptoms that can include insomnia or sleeping too many hours during the day, loss of appetite, or a very low activity level. Unlike the anxiety disorders, which often appear during childhood, most cases of depression do not emerge until adolescence or the adult years. Depression during childhood may have distinctive causes because the drugs that help depressed adults are less effective with children. The highest incidence of depression among Europeans and Americans occurs during the third decade, when adults are dealing with the stress of establishing a career and raising young children. Some cases of depression occur only during the winter months, when the hours of daylight are reduced. Many of these patients are helped by daily exposure to an hour of blue light, which has an excitatory effect on the brain.

Although the probability of suicide by a depressed patient is extremely low (less than 1 in 1,000), and more women than men make an attempt, more men actually take their lives, in part because men have easier access to guns. But even the probability of this rare act by an American adolescent is influenced by a combinations of social class and ethnicity (a little more frequent among higher-income African American adolescents than among those from economically disadvantaged homes), region (more likely in less densely populated states), time of year (higher in spring and summer), and day of the week (highest on Mondays).

In his book *Understanding and Treating Depression*, Rudy Nydegger, a psychologist, presents the thoughts of a sixty-one-year-old man who inherited a temperamental bias for depression:

> The earliest I remember being depressed was in the third grade; my teacher said that I appeared to have a very lazy and negative attitude and decided to help me by punishing this obviously bad behavior. . . . At that moment I realized that how I felt was different from the other kids and that to be safe and to avoid punishment I needed to hide inside myself and suffer alone. . . . For me it seems an affliction I was born with, and the only blame I can lay is on faulty genes. . . . On both sides of my family depression was common. . . . When depressed, I have chronic sleep deprivation, a lack of motivation, feelings of despair, a bizarre diet, social isolation, paranoid feelings, and at the end of an episode the blackness—nothing, a void. . . . While depressed I suffer mysterious aches and pains, gastric problems, neglected hygiene, and the aggravation of chronic pain from earlier injuries. . . . Professionally, I am a composer of classical music and need my mind and wits about me in the most complete manner possible. When depressed, the symptoms make it impossible for me to work, but when on medication I find that after a while I find my mental acuity and creativity blunted. . . . What I need to do is to catch the depression before it gets too bad and start on the medication (pp. 17–19).

As with most anxiety disorders, most depressions require a temperamental bias, a particular childhood history, and a set of current circumstances that precipitates the change in mood. A review of many studies reveals that most of the attempts to link a gene and a set of life events to an increased risk for depression have been unsuccessful because there are different biological and experiential causes of this symptom. For example, youth and young adults who had both a depressed parent and a depressed grandparent were at risk for developing social phobia or panic disorder rather than depression. A few investigators reported that possession of the short allele in the promoter region of the gene for the serotonin transporter molecule combined with a history of life adversity placed an adult at higher risk for depression. Unfortunately, many later studies failed to support this claim, although a history of adversity, without this or any other allele, increases the probability of developing a bout of depression.

However, the early reports of a causal relation between the combination of this allele and adversity, on the one hand, and the onset of a depression, on the other, can be understood if those with the short allele were temperamentally susceptible to exaggerating the emotional salience of a stressful event, such as loss of a love relationship, school or job failure, or social rejection. If those with the long allele who encountered the same unpleasant events did not experience them as unusually stressful, they would not mention them when a questionnaire asked them to list the adverse events of the past few years. If this suggestion is true, there would be a relation between possession of the short allele plus adversity and an increased risk for depression, but it would be a result of the person's exaggerated response to an unpleasant event rather than to the objective frequency of stressful events. A second reason for the inconsistent relation between possession of this allele and depression is that some individuals who have the short allele for the serotonin transporter inherit another gene that mitigates its effects on the brain.

Nonetheless, it is likely that there are alleles, as yet undiscovered, that do render a person vulnerable to a serious depression. This guess is based on the fact that the molecule dopamine (mentioned in chapter 4) is critical for the enthusiasm that is required to work for months or years toward a goal that is difficult to obtain. Dopamine excites a structure (the nucleus accumbens) that is a critical component of a circuit that motivates animals to approach a wanted object, such as food or water. Thus it is reasonable to assume that alleles that impair the secretion of dopamine, or reduce the density of its receptors, will dilute the psychological state that prompts humans to begin each day with the hope that something good might happen. Without that feeling there is no reason to greet the morning with more than the apathy that is a sign of depression. It appears that humans need to feel a minimal level of arousal, which some might call vitality, in order to commit energy to their responsibilities and remain loyal to their ethical standards. Depending on the person's history and culture, the targets of commitment can be a romantic partner, family members, religion, work, hobby, ideological cause, or increased wealth, fame, or power. The level of passion invested in pursuit of any of these goals usually becomes diluted during the later years, partly because of the reduced secretion of dopamine. This is one reason why depressed patients treated with drugs who improve temporarily often suffer a depression later in life, especially if they are poor or have become victims of the common illnesses of old age.

Family 3

McHugh's third family includes patients who are addicted to drugs, alcohol, or gambling, those who find it difficult to inhibit their sexual or aggressive urges, and those who cannot sustain attention in situations, like a school setting, where concentration is adaptive. These symptoms are more common among males than females, in part because men are more likely than women to turn to alcohol or drugs when they feel anxious or unhappy. Any one of these symptoms can be the product of different biological profiles. For example, different neurochemical mechanisms are responsible for the pleasure derived from cocaine, amphetamine, heroin, alcohol, cigarettes, or marijuana. However, most individuals in family 3 do not initially show the serious compromises in perception, reasoning, memory, language, or consciousness that characterize those in family 1.

Despite the extraordinary diversity of causes and symptoms characterizing the illnesses of family 3, many patients show compromised functioning of the prefrontal cortex, a site that facilitates the inhibition of inappropriate behavior. The genes and molecules that affect the integrity of the prefrontal cortex differ from those that have a major influence on the amygdala and the insula. The latter structures, which contribute to emotions, are more often implicated in the symptoms of family 2 illnesses. In one study, when hungry adults were told to inhibit their desire for food while looking at and tasting the foods they most liked, a majority reported feeling less hungry, and the brain areas normally activated by the sight of tasty food became less active.

This fact implies that the psychological process that the nineteenth century called willpower involves select brain sites that moderate the link between desire and action. Most humans are not helpless victims of their biology. A majority of rapists, pedophiles, and murderers have the ability to control their cruel behavior and, therefore, are not completely blameless. William Alanson

White, an eminent psychiatrist, and Bernard Glueck, an expert on crime, told a Chicago jury in 1924 that Richard Loeb and Nathan Leopold, two privileged young adults who had murdered an adolescent boy to prove they could commit a crime and remain undiscovered, were insane and not totally responsible for their crime. However, the jury, in its wisdom, found both men guilty and sent them to prison.

ADHD

Some, but not all, children and adults with attention-deficit/hyperactivity disorder possess a compromise in the integrity of the prefrontal cortex. This diagnosis is being given more often by physicians in North America and Europe, approaching 5 to 10 percent of all children, with three times as many boys as girls receiving this label. Children are classified as having ADHD if they (1) find it difficult to sustain attention on a task requiring concentration, (2) are excessively restless, or (3) are unusually impulsive. Each of these characteristics can occur without the others, and each can be the result of different combinations of biology and life experience. The impulsivity or restlessness is more often due to compromises in dopamine activity, but impaired attention can be the result of compromises in the activity of the molecule acetylcholine. Thus, the category ADHD includes different kinds of patients. The heritability of this diagnosed condition is modest—identical twins are only a little more likely than non-identical twins to be assigned this diagnostic label. There is even evidence to suggest that the causes of ADHD in males might differ from the causal profiles in females.

Although scientists believe that a large proportion of ADHD patients suffer from an abnormality in dopamine functioning, it has been difficult to prove this conjecture beyond doubt, despite the fact that the drug usually prescribed, called Ritalin, increases dopamine activity in the frontal lobe. One reason for this frustration is that the level of dopamine activity in varied brain sites is influenced by a host of independent factors, including the amount of dopamine secreted by neurons in the brain stem, the effects of dopamine on neurons in the outer shell of the nucleus accumbens, and the activity level of two molecules that reduce the amount of dopamine in the synapses. Each of these factors is controlled by different alleles. Thus a person could possess the allele for one molecule that led to the rapid reduction of dopamine in the brain's synapses along with the allele for another molecule that reduced dopamine activity more slowly. This complexity makes it difficult for scientists to predict the actual level of dopamine activity in a particular brain location. It is reasonable, however, to expect that future research will reveal that some form of abnormal dopamine activity contributes to ADHD symptoms in some patients.

Conduct disorder and bulimia

The children who are consistently disobedient and the youths or adults who are addicted to alcohol or drugs or engage in binge eating followed by self-induced vomiting, called bulimics, find it difficult to control their maladaptive urges. Most patients with bulimia do not show the extreme degree of self-control that is characteristic of anorexics. This fact implies that anorexia and bulimia may be the product of different temperamental biases and life histories, even though the psychiatrists' habit of classifying both symptoms as "eating disorders" tempts investigators to search for a common set of causal conditions.

The influence of history

The symptoms that define the illnesses of family 3 are subject to increases or decreases in prevalence over time because some of the symptoms that define the category depend on the values of the local society, and these values change over time. For example, a World Health Organization study found that sex differences in the abuse of alcohol and drugs among adults in fifteen countries was smaller among eighteen-to-thirty-four-year-olds than among those over age sixty-five because of historical events that made it more acceptable for younger women to abuse these substances. Frequent drinking to intoxication is characteristic of a small proportion of individuals in every society that learned how to make beer, wine, or spirits. I noted in chapter 5 that individuals who possess alleles that slow the activity of the enzymes that metabolize alcohol, more often Caucasians and Africans than Asians, are at a higher risk for becoming alcoholic. However, most older societies did not regard such individuals as mentally ill. Neither Hippocrates nor Galen posited any temperamental type as the origin of alcoholism.

Felicia Huppert of Cambridge University notes that if a behavior is much more common in one small region of a society, then citizens in the larger society are tempted to regard the deviant trait as a mental illness. For example, in thirty-two different countries there was an almost perfect relation between the average amount of alcohol consumed by residents living in one particular region and the proportion who were classified by professionals as alcohol addicts in need of medical treatment.

Americans in 1830 regarded the heavy consumption of alcohol and prostitution as moral failures, not as mental illnesses, and, then as now, both habits were more common among the less well educated. The middle-class Americans who tried to reform alcoholics by advocating temperance movements several times over the past 175 years believed, correctly, that changes in the environment could have therapeutic consequences. If we improved the quality of the schools attended by children of impoverished families, we might reduce the incidence of the mental illnesses in family 3, and perhaps those in family 2 as well, by a considerable amount.

The main point is that historical and cultural conditions, and their associated ethical values, exert a far greater influence on the prevalence and evaluation of the seriousness of the symptoms in family 3 than in the first two families. This claim is obvious for homicide. Mothers in many parts of the economically less-developed world kill their newborn infants if they cannot feed them. In parts of south India some mothers kill their infant daughters if they are certain that they will be unable to afford a dowry when the girl is ready to marry. None of these mothers is regarded as mentally ill by their society, but most would be declared criminally insane if they lived in the United States. Americans would classify a middle-class accountant who strapped explosives around his waist and blew himself up in a Los Angeles shopping mall as mentally ill. However, a college-educated Palestinian who committed the same act in a restaurant in Haifa would be celebrated by his village and proclaimed a heroic martyr, as were the eleventh-century crusaders who died while slaughtering Muslims in Jerusalem.

Although the Don Juan in Mozart's opera was selfish, uncontrolled, and emotionally callous, he was not considered mentally ill. A homosexual lifestyle, which had been regarded as a crime and a sign of mental illness in the nineteenth century, was cleansed of all taint by a vote of the American Psychiatric Association, despite the absence of any new scientific evidence. The change in the psychiatric status of a gay adult by committee vote implies that the classification of a behavior as a sign of mental illness can, on occasion, depend on the values of a society. Most psychiatrists would classify a thirty-five-year-old chronic liar who felt no empathy for others as a psychopath. However, the many employees of banks and mortgage companies who persuaded poor families to borrow large amounts of money that they knew the families could not repay were also callously dishonest. In that case, however, psychiatrists would be less confident in diagnosing them as psychopaths because their actions were legitimate in our economy. Thus the bases for the deviant behaviors that harm others differ from the causes of the deviant features that define the categories of family 1. Every society, ancient and modern, would agree that anyone who could not carry on coherent conversations, banged his head against a wall, was unable to remember what had happened an hour earlier, or wandered aimlessly down a street yelling obscenities must be mentally disturbed.

Family 4

McHugh's fourth family is unique because the symptoms, usually those of families 2 or 3, are attributable only to the person's life history and current social conditions and do not require a special biological vulnerability. The usual circumstances that lead to anxiety, depression, school failure, substance abuse, or antisocial behavior include a history of child abuse, a life of poverty, or parents who failed to encourage school achievement and to discourage aggression and impulsivity. These symptoms are more common among the poor and marginalized in every society. There is, however, one potential advantage of a deprived or harsh childhood. If people from such backgrounds are able to combine talent, perseverance, and a little luck to achieve a satisfying job and/or a stable marriage, they are apt to feel chronically happy because they will compare their current state with the sadness and worry that pervaded their childhood years.

The brain reacts to an aversive event, whether pain, failure, or loss, by activating a cluster of neurons, called the rostromedial tegmental nucleus, that temporarily suppresses a site that secretes dopamine. Recall that the surge of dopamine to an unexpected event that was desired contributes to a brief feeling of pleasure. It is possible that continued poverty, neglect, rejection, failure, or marginalization can lead to a chronic reduction of dopamine secretion and create a cynical, dour personality that has difficulty experiencing the pleasure or excitement that accompanies the anticipation of a wished-for event.

A pre-adolescent girl from Newcastle-on-Tyne in England killed two small preschool boys in 1968 for no apparent reason. The girl's father was a criminal, and her mother, a prostitute, forced her four-year-old daughter to perform fellatio on her clients. She told a writer many years later that her horrific childhood experiences led her to conclude that she was fundamentally a bad person who deserved to be punished. The murder of the boys accomplished two goals—it affirmed her categorization of self as bad and, simultaneously, provided the community with a reason to punish her.

Brief periods of worry, a phobia, nightmares, or apathy occur to many children, adolescents, and adults and do not always become chronic symptoms. Many children suffer from nightmares for several days after watching a horror film. One of my students, now a well-adjusted faculty member at a major university, developed a phobia of birds that lasted for a few years after seeing Hitchcock's film *The Birds* because, as a child, she regarded birds as gentle and beautiful. The film's depiction of birds as dangerous was a sufficiently serious violation of her belief to create a state of uncertainty that led to the temporary phobia.

I developed a phobia of films containing scenes of blood on victims of violence that lasted for a little less than two years. After checking into a hotel in Nashville at about 6 p.m. on April 4, 1968, I turned on the television set and learned that Martin Luther King had been assassinated. The unique state of my body and mind, created by the combination of no dinner and a blend of surprise, anger, and sadness, motivated me to leave the room and take a walk. An hour later I found myself in downtown Nashville looking up at a marquee advertising the film *Bonnie and Clyde*. My students had recommended the movie and, needing distraction, I went in and sat down at the moment, toward the end of the film, when Bonnie and Clyde are trapped in their car and being fired on by police. As blood appeared on their faces I felt faint. I got up and walked to the lobby, where I fell to the floor unconscious for a few minutes. I have very low blood pressure and was vulnerable to this reaction. After regaining consciousness, I returned to the hotel. But I did not realize at the time that this brief experience, combined with fatigue from the trip and the emotional distress over King's murder, had established a classically conditioned fainting response to the sight of blood shown as a result of an inflicted injury in a movie or on television. I avoided all such films until the conditioned response vanished spontaneously about eighteen months later. This phobia would not have developed if I had not been emotionally upset by the assassination, and it did not extend to the sight of blood on my body or the body of another if it was not caused by violence. I did not seek help from a psychiatrist because I thought I understood the reason for the symptom, and it did not interfere with my responsibilities or generally good mood. Had I gone to a doctor I would have been classified as a blood phobic and added to the published statistics on this "illness."

There are many thousands of similar cases in every country. Older adults who have learned that they do not sleep well if they drink regular coffee after dinner avoid this drink and substitute herbal tea. But they are not classified as possessing a coffee phobia. Once we understand the physiological basis for the uncomfortable feeling that some adults experience when they look out from a tall building or a high cliff, this reaction, too, may be dropped from the list of mental illnesses, as long as it does not interfere with performing the tasks of the day and is restricted to a particular situation.

Measures of the brain might be able to discriminate between a bout of depression that belongs to family 2 and one belonging to family 4. Depressed patients who show greater activity in the frontal lobe of the right hemisphere, compared with the left, are usually not helped by modern drugs, whereas those who show greater activity in the frontal lobe in the left hemisphere do profit from the drug treatment. It is possible that some of the former patients belong to family 2 and some of the latter to family 4.

Loretta Cass and Carolyn Thomas conducted a forgotten but important long-term study that began in the 1950s that has implications for our understanding of the consequences of a mental illness in children. A group of about two hundred mainly working-class mothers living in St. Louis were troubled by the behaviors of their children, who ranged in age from six to fifteen years, and brought them to a local clinic. There were three times as many boys as girls, and two-thirds of the youngsters were either failing in school or were extremely disobedient. Only one in five was unusually shy and fearful. Six to fifteen years later, when some of these former child patients were in their third decade, psychiatrists and psychologists interviewed them. The findings surprised Cass and Thomas, but would be less surprising to contemporary psychiatrists and clinical psychologists. The vast majority were adjusting to the demands of their society, implying that all children try to use their benevolent experiences to grow toward better health. The 19 percent who were still seriously disturbed had been the most labile infants and the most impulsive children (temperament), were born to less-well-educated parents with lower incomes (social class), and were more often later-borns rather than firstborns. Thus temperament, social class, and birth order all contributed to the persistence of the earlier symptoms.

The Pattern Is Primary

It is worth repeating that frequent bouts of anxiety or depression can occur in patients belonging to any one of McHugh's four families and can be the product of different combinations of genes, temperaments, cultural backgrounds, and life histories. For example, a bipolar patient from family 1, an anxious adolescent from family 2, a drug addict from family 3, and a poor, unemployed Hispanic mother from family 4 can all experience a serious depression or a combination of depression and anxiety. Therefore, the presence of these emotions, even when intense, does not distinguish among the different categories of mental illness. These emotional states, when considered alone, rather than as elements in a pattern of features, are analogous to the color of a surface. Some cauliflowers, horses, roses, and picket fences are white.

It is also important to appreciate that the sharp rise in diagnoses of mental illness in children during the past twenty-five years is partly due to the fact that the parents of these children worry about their academic progress and can obtain special resources that would not be forthcoming if the child were called retarded, incorrigible, or unmotivated rather than autistic, bipolar, or learning disabled. The economies in many parts of the developed world require every child to complete high school with adequate language and mathematical skills and to go on to receive a college degree if he or she wishes to obtain a job with financial security and dignity. Hence, children who cannot meet these criteria are at risk for becoming anxious, depressed, alcoholic, drug-addicted, or criminal. A college diploma was not a requirement for successful adjustment in the eighteenth century; Benjamin Franklin did not have the advantage of even three years of formal education.

Contemporary middle-class youth in North America and most of Europe are vulnerable to brief bouts of anxiety or apathy because of the unique historical events of the past half century. These events include the requirement to be tolerant of people advocating any value system or displaying a practice, no matter how unusual, as long as it is not harmful to others. These conditions make it difficult for youth to commit passion to the defeat of a morally abhorrent ideology. Many young adults have no cause to fight for other than maximizing their pleasure, getting good grades, acquiring more friends, and obtaining a higher status.

Moreover, the absence of serious suffering among most who were raised in middle-class families provokes a little guilt because these privileged youth are aware of the plight of many adults in nations with low income levels or in refugee camps in Darfur, Congo, and Rwanda. This combination of facts probably contributes to rates of suicide, self-mutilation, and drug addiction that are considerably higher than those recorded a half century ago. The creation of community service programs in many high schools may be helpful.

American adolescents reared by conservative religious families that regarded atheism and a gay lifestyle as morally wrong might begin to question the validity of the values they have regarded as permanently true after interacting with peers who hold more liberal views. For example, they might begin to wonder about the moral necessity of honesty and loyalty if the courts insist that atheists and gays are entitled to equal dignity. This questioning of childhood ethical beliefs can be accompanied by some uncertainty about their sense of virtue because of the challenge to their former ethical position.

The American ethic demanding tolerance and egalitarianism, which obligates each citizen to award equal dignity to everyone no matter what their values or behaviors, has contributed to the attractiveness of the idea that most mental illnesses are due to a specific biological cause. This ethic makes it politically incorrect to insist that parents make a contribution to the poor academic performance or aggressive behavior of some children, and easy to argue that genes are usually the primary culprit. The latter perspective removes much of the blame from both the person and his or her family for the unfortunate state of the former. To be labeled mentally ill in this century bears some resemblance to the state of an innocent fifteenth-century victim of a malevolent witch.

The benevolent social gains that are the result of our egalitarian ethos, which I celebrate, have exacted a small cost—there are no free lunches. The availability of technologies that can detect genes, along with the media's hyping of biological determinism, have persuaded many Americans and Europeans that genes and the temperamental biases they create must be exceedingly potent causes of mental illness, even though no team of scientists has found any particular gene or cluster of genes that is a consistent correlate of poor attention skills, hyperactivity, aggressive behavior, academic failure, chronic disobedience, depression, or anxiety that is independent of the person's gender, social class, ethnicity, cultural background, and unique pattern of life experiences.

7

What Have We Learned?

Every person is born with a unique biology and pattern of temperamental biases. Even identical twins who have the same genes on the day of their conception are not identical in every feature on the day of their birth nine months later because of chance events affecting only one of the fetuses during the prenatal months. The probability that any two individuals from different family pedigrees will share the same set of eight genes is less than eight in one hundred million million, which implies that such a coincidence is close to impossible. The more significant fact is that many of the behaviors that appear to be temperamental biases, such as irritability, smiling, or restlessness, can have more than one origin. Therefore, it is useful to adopt McHugh's strategy and parse the large number of biases into a small number of categories that share critical features.

A Set of Temperamental Categories

One strategy for categorizing the large number of human temperaments relies on three criteria: (1) Is the bias due primarily to a chemical profile in the brain or some feature of brain anatomy? (2) Is the bias due to a heritable set of alleles or the result of prenatal or early postnatal events? and, finally, (3) Does the biological foundation of the temperament influence primarily the limbic parts of the brain, which are closely associated with emotional excitability, or sites in the frontal lobe, which are more important in the regulation of impulsive behavior? Eight temperamental types are possible if we divide each feature into two parts and ask whether the bias is primarily neurochemical or neuroanatomical, inherited or not inherited, and affecting emotional excitability or impulsive behavior (table 1).

	Neurochemical		Neuroanatomical	
	Inherited	Not Inherited	Inherited	Not Inherited
Excite Emotion	1	2	3	4
Control Impulse	5	6	7	8

Table 1.

The high- and low-reactive infants described in chapter 2 would be assigned to cell 1 (a neurochemical origin, inherited, and affecting emotional excitability). The temperament that Mary Rothbart called regulation would be assigned to cell 5 (neurochemical, inherited, and related to the control of impulsive behavior). Some children diagnosed with ADHD or conduct disorder would also be in cell 5, but others belong to cells 6, 7, or 8. Of course, the individuals who acquired a diagnosis of social anxiety or ADHD without any special biology do not belong to any of the eight cells. The research task is to fill in descriptions of the temperamental types that belong to each of the eight cells by gathering biological evidence, test performance results, and behavioral observations in natural settings. When this goal is achieved, pharmaceutical companies might develop drugs tailored to the particular temperament of a depressed or anxious patient. Perhaps even psychotherapists will accommodate to the specific temperamental or experiential origin of a symptom.

One of the most serious frustrations is our inability to detect the temperamental biases of adults with varied personalities because we do not know which genes or molecules contributed to their adult profile. At present, the pattern of temperamental biases possessed by an adult is analogous to a drop of black ink that has been dissolved in a glass of glycerin and is no longer visible.

We also do not know the range of behavioral and emotional reactions of the individuals in a particular cell, nor the degree to which social class, gender, ethnicity, and life experience influence their adult profiles. It is unlikely, at least for the foreseeable future, that any expert will be able to tell parents with certainty that their newborn infant inherited an uncommon temperament. When an inherited physical disease is rare, say an incidence of less than one in one thousand, the current biological test for the disease makes too many errors because rare events are difficult to predict. For example, if every one of the approximately 4 million American infants born in 2009 were tested for any of the fifty rare diseases mediated by a single known gene, the test would be incorrect 98 percent of the time. The result of the test would indicate that about twelve hundred newborns had the disease, when in fact only eighteen would actually develop the symptoms.

Social Class

It is worth repeating the message in chapter 3 that the social class in which a child is reared exerts a profound influence on the adult outcomes of the temperaments associated with any of the eight cells. The members of every society vary in power, status, wealth, or privilege. Those who believe they have less privilege are a little more vulnerable to anxiety, envy, anger, self-doubt, or a blend of two or more of these emotions.

Robert Nozick, a distinguished Harvard philosopher who grew up in a poor, immigrant Jewish family, questioned his right to think about profound intellectual themes, once writing: "Isn't it ludicrous for someone just one generation from the shtetl, a pisher from Brownsville and East Flatbush in Brooklyn, even to touch on the topics of the monumental thinkers?" Bertrand Russell, who spent his childhood in a privileged family, would not have harbored such doubts.

The higher prevalence of the mental illnesses in McHugh's families 2, 3, or 4 (due to a serious brain abnormality, a temperamental bias for anxiety or depression, or a bias affecting regulation of behavior) among the economically disadvantaged is exacerbated if there is unusually high income inequality in a city or region. Social class can even compete with the effects of child abuse. Children who suffered serious abuse or neglect were at a higher risk for depression than most, but the risk was almost as large (21 vs. 25 percent) for those growing up in a disadvantaged-class category who were neither abused nor neglected. This fact does not mean that childhood abuse is unimportant; rather, it implies that the experiences and identifications that are linked to one's social class have a powerful effect on adult moods. Social class also predicts the probability of recovery following psychiatric treatment. Drugs or psychotherapy are a little less likely to help impoverished patients with an anxiety disorder than middle-class patients with the same complaints.

The majority of youths who have been arrested for a crime or diagnosed as learning disabled come from families in the bottom third of the income distribution who live in poor neighborhoods and attend inadequate schools. We usually treat these adolescents with drugs rather than spending the money to improve their schools and neighborhoods or hiring tutors for struggling students. If a section of a large city reported an unusually high incidence of diarrhea, public health officials would clean up the water supply rather than treat each patient with medicine each time he or she became ill.

Surprisingly, a person's voice is affected by the status of the individual with whom they are interacting, even though they have no conscious awareness of these changes. Two scientists analyzed the speech samples from twenty-five different interviews that Larry King, a television talk show host, conducted with varied guests. When King was talking with a person of high status—for example, Bill Clinton—he began to match the pitch, loudness, and rhythm of his voice to that of his guest. However, when King was interviewing less eminent individuals—for example, Dan Quayle—the guests began to match their voices to King's.

Membership in a class category creates boundaries that restrict the range of possible actions, intentions, and emotional responses, as an enclosure restricts the movements of a herd of cows. Although most youths know there are successful musicians in symphony orchestras and physicists in universities, the proportion of poor adolescents who believe they can become professional cellists or astrophysicists is smaller than the proportion found among advantaged youth. And fewer economically privileged adolescents consider becoming professional boxers or football players.

The variation among the fourteen types of finches scattered across the Galapagos Islands provides an analogy. Although the fourteen types differ in coloration, size, and shape of beak, all of which are heritable, they also differ in the song the male sings, which affects his eventual mating partner. However, the subtle features that distinguish the songs of the fourteen species are not inherited; they are learned early in development. Similarly, humans growing up in different class groups are exposed to distinctive experiences and educational opportunities that affect their choice of vocation and spouse. Fortunately, the barriers between the advantaged and the disadvantaged in human societies are more porous than the ecological barriers that separate the varied types of finches.

History and Culture

The historical era and culture in which a life is lived also shape the psyches of those with distinctive temperaments. The historical changes that brought technologies, public education, and economies based on information, rather than crops or manufacturing, have created unique constellations of beliefs, values, and emotions that were not possible when the Egyptians built the pyramids. The feeling of alienation experienced by some Iraqi immigrants living in Los Angeles and the emotion felt by sixth-century Mayans watching a young maiden being thrown down a deep well in order to please the god that brought rain are distinctive states evoked in those living in particular cultures at a particular time. The themes of the cartoons in the *New Yorker* magazine from 1929 to the present reveal historical changes in the ideas that troubled the middle-class readers of this magazine. The cartoons from 1929 to 1955 satirized the idle rich, Ivy League graduates, and older men seducing younger women. The targets of satire from 1955 to the present, which would have been regarded as offensive in 1929, were female self-interest, the boredom of work, the dubious value of higher education, and the ennui and spiritual emptiness of modern life. A 1992 cartoon illustrated a corral holding a large group of well-dressed young men and a man outside the corral saying, "In 6 weeks these MBAs will be ready for market." Another depicted a woman entering a house after placing three boxes of recyclable garbage on the sidewalk. Two boxes contained old bottles and paper; the third held a man.

The nineteenth-century diarist Alice James and the novelist John Cheever probably inherited the same temperamental bias for melancholic moods. However, each of these writers imposed a different interpretation on their depression because of the historical era in which each one lived. Cheever, who was born in 1912 and was influenced by Freudian ideas, assumed that his melancholy was traceable to early experiences in the family. Alice James, born in 1848, eight years before Freud's birth, was convinced that she had inherited her depressive moods and did not blame her parents' actions for her unhappiness. Three distinct personalities would emerge if a woman with Alice James's temperament grew up in (1) a seventeenth-century Puritan New England town, (2) a village in medieval France, or (3) contemporary Chicago.

I was one of many speakers at a scientific conference in Washington, D.C., about twenty years ago. Following my presentation on temperament, an older biologist gave the last talk of the morning and after returning to his seat, he asked if we could have lunch together. We found a small restaurant away from the crowd where he told me that my talk had changed his understanding of his extreme vulnerability to anxiety. He had been an extremely shy boy and an introverted adolescent, and he continued to experience intense anxiety before making a presentation to an audience. Like Cheever, he had always assumed that his emotional vulnerability was created by the practices and personality of his parents. My evidence had persuaded him of the flaw in that explanation, and he was ready to acknowledge that he had probably inherited a temperament similar to the one possessed by high-reactive infants. Because interpretations of private feelings affect moods and behaviors, this biologist's new insight probably reduced his anger at his family and perhaps created a more serene acceptance of his vulnerability to uncertainty when speaking to large audiences.

Historical events make it easy or difficult for people with particular temperaments to adjust to their community. The changes over the past eight thousand years that have obvious implications for the temperaments of high and low reactivity include: (1) the greater emphasis on the solitary individual seeking gratification compared with reliance on one's family and social group, (2) the need to interact with many strangers, (3) the need to compete with peers, and (4) the relative advantage of taking risks over adopting a risk-averse style. These conditions have made it harder for high-reactives and easier for low-reactives to cope with the demands of their community. Perhaps that is why there are twice as many low- as high-reactive infants among Caucasian populations. Finches on one of the Galapagos Islands who inherited large beaks increased in numbers while those with small beaks decreased after climate changes produced more large seeds that were harder to crack for finches with small beaks.

However, the contemporary hyping of the power of genes to create anxious and depressed moods may have muted the intensity of guilt felt by those with high-reactive temperaments when they betrayed a friend or brooded on their personal contribution to their timidity. The same historical narrative has made it easier for those with a low-reactive temperament to become more callous, selfish, and aggressive than those with the same temperament born several centuries earlier. The account is balanced; high-reactives feel a little less responsible for their chronic tension, but low-reactives are a little more dangerous. The main point is that neither a high- nor a low-reactive temperament is always better adapted; rather, the advantages of each bias depend on the local culture.

Gender

It is useful to restate the important contribution of temperament to the sculpting of a person's conception of his or her gender. Modern screenwriters agree with the ancient Greek playwrights that women prefer acts of love to waging war. This idea, deeply embedded in the unconscious of most women, makes it difficult for them to be extremely violent or cruel. Men committed most of the murders in Hitler's Germany, Stalin's Soviet Union, and the villages in Rwanda, Bosnia, Sri Lanka, and Sudan. I suspect that more Americans were shocked by seeing the photographs of a woman torturing an Iraqi prisoner than those who saw the photos of male soldiers engaged in the same shameful behavior. The excess number of murders committed by men is not simply the result of male hormone, but is partly the product of unconscious representations of the actions that males believe they have a license to display. Shakespeare had Lady Macbeth ask to be "unsexed" so she could participate in the murder of the king.

I suggested in chapter 4 that many children and adults possess an unconscious symbolic network that links the concept of female with the concept of nature. As a result, the features that are appropriate for females often vary with whether the society views nature as harsh or gentle, predictable or uncontrollable, a source of beauty or a source of danger. If citizens believe that labile emotional displays are closer to nature's intention than a subdued persona, women will be characterized as unpredictably emotional. If, on the other hand, reason is nature's preferred plan, women will be regarded as scheming and cunning. Most contemporary Americans and Europeans believe that they should be loyal to the Darwinian principle that all animals are concerned primarily with their survival and welfare. As a result, contemporary biologists describe females as self-interested when they choose or separate from a mate. A *New Yorker* cartoon illustrated a middle-aged couple listening to a lawyer read from a document: "The wife gets the house, the car, the dog, the I.R.A., and $10,000 a month. In return, she acknowledges your right to exist."

The varied combinations of biology and culture create slightly different states of consciousness in males and females. The small number of men who request surgery to become females experience a passivity that contrasts with the feeling of active intrusiveness that characterizes the typical masculine approach to challenge and sexuality. The evidence implies, but has not yet proven, that men and women experience slightly different psychological states when interacting, or planning an interaction, with a love object, family member, or friend. A pair of Princeton University scientists asked men and women from a variety of social classes about their sexual motives and satisfactions. More females than males said that enhancing the pleasure of their partner was an important motive. More males than females said that they wanted the satisfaction of knowing that they had been potent lovers. A speculative abstraction from all the evidence suggests that more females than males want to know that others need their love and kindness and feel gratitude toward them for the ministrations of these resources. More males than females want to know that others will defer to them and acknowledge their potency.

Few male poets could have written the following lines from an Emily Dickinson poem:

My river runs to thee:
Blue sea, wilt welcome me?

. . . .

Say, sea,
Take me!

By contrast, it is unlikely that a thirteenth-century female poet would have written these lines from a poem by Rumi:

Think that you're gliding not from the face of a cliff
like an eagle. Think you're walking
like a tiger walks by himself in the forest.

What Can Be Changed?

Our studies of high- and low-reactive infants taught us that both types of adolescents found it relatively easy to alter how they appeared to others—this is the public face that Jung called the persona. However, high-reactive adolescents found it far more difficult to control their continued vulnerability to pangs of worry over an unexpected event that they could not immediately understand. Most psychotherapists can help patients who are afraid of flying to board an airplane and sit through the flight, but they are less successful in preventing a feeling of tension rising as the plane taxis on the runway; it is easier to change behaviors that are under voluntary control than to alter feelings that arise spontaneously. Humans can learn to approach objects or places that are feared, but are less able to change their feelings. That is why phobias have always been the easiest symptoms to cure. Oscar (from the film *The Odd Couple*) could probably have persuaded Felix to behave less compulsively when he cleaned their apartment, but he would have been less successful in preventing Felix from worrying when the evening news predicted a serious snowstorm. A cartoon in the *New Yorker* illustrated a despondent man sitting by an open window where a bluebird, which has alighted on the sill, tells the hapless man, "Happiness is not readily transmittable from bluebirds to humans."

In every mammalian species some animals are bold; some are timid. For example, bold guppies approach large, unfamiliar fish that are potential predators, whereas timid guppies stay away. Although the possession of a bold temperament has the serious disadvantage of increasing the risk of being eaten, it turns out that female guppies prefer to mate with the bold rather than the timid males. Introverts miss the joys that come from meeting new people and visiting new places but have the advantage of living a few years longer than extroverts.

Effective political leaders must be able to suppress the guilt that follows violation of a personal moral standard if the standard is incompatible with the nation's best interests. Only some temperaments permit this suppression. When a reporter asked Pierre Mendes-France, a former leader of France, what qualities were required in a great statesman, Mendes-France was probably thinking of Franklin Delano Roosevelt when he replied, "They should not be too sentimental." Stephen Daedalus, the hero in Joyce's *Portrait of the Artist as a Young Man*, who refused to go to Easter Mass to please his mother because to do so required him to violate his skeptical view of religion and render him vulnerable to guilt, would not have been a great president or prime minister.

Temperament and Morality

Temperaments contribute to the substantial variation in the intensity of the anxiety, shame, or guilt that can accompany the contemplation or commission of an action that violates a personal or community standard. Although parental socialization always influences the degree of restraint imposed on asocial behaviors, each person's temperament remains potent. Antonio Damasio, an eminent neuroscientist who has written about emotions, described a man who lost the ventromedial surface of his prefrontal cortex as a result of surgery. Although he had been intelligent and successful prior to surgery, he suddenly began to make impulsive decisions, despite no change in his measured intelligence.

One reason was that this part of the brain receives information from the amygdala, which milliseconds earlier had received inputs from the heart, lung, gut, and muscles via neurons in the medulla. A person without a ventromedial surface cannot experience the subtle feeling that most of us experience when we have the urge to risk a large amount of money in the stock market or to move from friends and family to a distant location for a better job. Recall from chapter 2 that the eighteen-year-old high-reactives, who experience an unusually salient feeling of uncertainty after a mistake, had a thicker cortex than low-reactives in a small part of the right ventromedial cortical surface.

I suggested in chapter 1 that infants vary in the intensity of the unpleasant feeling produced by a pain or a bitter taste, as well as in the intensity of the pleasant feeling evoked by a sweet taste or a caress. It is possible that the variation among infants in the intensity of the pleasure or pain that accompanies different sensory experiences is preserved and applied to symbolic events later in life, such as the intensity of pride felt after completing a difficult task or the intensity of guilt following a mistake. This speculation rests on the discovery that some of the same brain structures (the anterior cingulate and insula) that are active in physical pain are also active when a person is rejected or loses some money. Analogously, some of the structures that are active when a person tastes an unexpectedly sweet food are active when the person is praised, especially the ventral tegmentum (a major source of dopamine), the nucleus accumbens, and the amygdala (figure 7). Should this bold suggestion prove correct, infants with a temperamental bias that amplified the discomfort felt by the prick of a diaper pin or a bitter taste might have a higher probability of becoming adolescents who were especially vulnerable to intense guilt following the violation of an ethical norm. And infants who laughed and babbled excitedly during a game of peekaboo might be a little more likely to become adults who experienced prolonged joy after receiving a gift they had wanted for months.

High-reactive adolescents are more certain of the actions they believe are absolutely right or wrong and find it easier to honor these imperatives in order to avoid corrosive feelings of guilt. Low-reactives, who find it easier to suspend absolute judgments of right and wrong, often adapt their ethical evaluation to local conditions. They may lie to a teacher but not to a friend. One low-reactive adolescent boy told an interviewer that he forged his parent's signature on a letter to the headmaster of a private school to which he had been accepted stating that the boy had decided

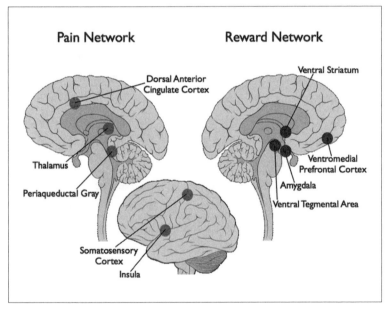

Figure 7. Illustration of the structures involved in the circuits that are usually activated by pain and reward.

not to attend the school. I cannot imagine a similar action from a high-reactive because the anticipated repercussions of the forgery would have provoked intensely uncomfortable feelings.

A woman examiner gave high- and low-reactive four-year-olds a color photograph of herself and said, "This is my favorite picture. Tear up my favorite picture." Most high-reactives became tense, looked at their mother, and afraid of disobeying the adult, tore off a small corner from the photograph. By contrast, most low-reactives tore the photo in half immediately, smiling as they did so, because in that setting that action seemed legitimate. One unusually bold low-reactive boy returned the photograph, saying, "No, it's your favorite picture. I won't do it." No high-reactive four-year-old would feel confident enough to refuse the adult's request. At age fifteen this boy told an interviewer that he was thinking about entering politics and running for president of the United States. I suspect that Bill Clinton had the same adolescent ambitions and am relatively certain that he was a low-reactive infant.

Carl Jung's recollection of a childhood incident illustrates the power of temperament to provoke a strong emotion when a moral standard is in jeopardy of being violated. On returning from school on an unusually lovely day, Jung recalls that he felt overwhelmed by the aesthetic pattern of light and shadow on a church roof. As he thought about the beauty of the scene and its source in God's actions, he suddenly experienced a numbness and an urge to stop thinking. "Don't go on thinking now. Something terrible is coming. Something I do not want to think, something I dare not approach." Jung remembers feeling afraid that he was about to have a sinful thought that would offend God.

High-reactives are vulnerable to a more intense guilt reaction to violations of moral beliefs than others because their more excitable amygdala creates higher levels of sympathetic activity that generate bodily sensations that are interpreted as guilt. The eleven-year-old high- and low-reactives described in chapter 2 ranked the degree to which each of twenty sentences described their personality. One sentence was, "I feel bad if one of my parents says that I did something wrong." High- and low-reactives had equivalent average ranks for that description. However, the high-reactives who endorsed this trait displayed more signs of amygdalar excitability than the low-reactives who also regarded this quality as a personal characteristic. This fact implies that the temperament of high-reactives renders them unusually vulnerable to strong emotion when they recognize an inconsistency between two beliefs or between a belief and their behavior. Low-reactives might recognize the inconsistency but it would bother them less. The ease with which the individual can adapt his or her evaluations and actions to the immediate setting represents a significant source of variation among humans.

Individuals who experience intense guilt about violations of a moral belief try to create strategies that might mute its corrosive consequences. I suspect that among the many married couples who quarrel continually, there is a small proportion in which one spouse with the temperament of a high-reactive is vulnerable to guilt over disloyalty to his or her moral standards. If these individuals sense that they have not met the expectations they suspect their partner holds for them, whether the invented obligation is greater sexual desire, affection toward a child, a higher income, an exceptional accomplishment, or a willingness to engage in the recreations the other likes, a feeling akin to guilt is generated. This guilt can arise even if the partner did not hold those expectations and the guilty spouse was not completely aware of being a less than satisfying husband or wife. A common reaction to the presumed failure is the adoption of a hostile, critical, or demanding demeanor in order to provoke the partner to retaliate and thereby reduce the uncomfortable feelings of the quarrelsome spouse. The boy called Amir in *The Kite Runner*, who cannot excise the disabling guilt he feels over not rescuing his loyal friend Hassan from an attack by three bullies, throws pomegranates at Hassan for no apparent reason in order to provoke a retaliation. A popular song of my youth was called, "You Always Hurt the One You Love." A similar dynamic occurs when a child who feels guilty over his or her failure to meet an affectionate parent's standard for school achievement becomes irrationally argumentative and disobedient. These children want to provoke a severe parental punishment so that they can label the parent as unreasonable and thereby rationalize their school failure and disobedience and, as a dividend, dilute their guilt. The authors of the Tree of Knowledge allegory in Genesis were exceptionally insightful when they had God tell Adam and Eve that their punishment for eating the apple was a continual awareness of right and wrong, which, out of kindness, He did not give to animals.

About one in four low-reactive boys possesses a unique temperament that is accompanied by extremely low levels of childhood fear, a more active left rather than right frontal lobe, and unusually low heart rate and blood pressure values. I suspect that these boys might become accomplished leaders if they grow up in homes with loving parents who encourage achievement and insist on the control of unprovoked aggression. However, if these same boys are raised by neglecting or indifferent parents and are exposed to criminal activity in their community, they are at risk for becoming delinquents or criminals. Antisocial ten-year-olds with very low heart rates and blood pressure are more likely to continue a criminal career into the adult years than equally delinquent children with higher heart rate and blood pressure values. The latter often give up their asocial habits during late adolescence. It is possible that a very small group of criminals who commit violent crimes year after year (probably less than 5 percent of all criminals) possess a rare temperament. A small number of New Zealand three- and five-year-old children, who were members of a longitudinal study in Dunedin, had great difficulty controlling impulsive, antisocial behavior. These atypical children were at the highest risk for becoming adults who committed one or more violent acts.

New Questions

The advantage of continued research is that unexpected discoveries force scientists to discard old questions that led to dead ends and to replace them with new ones. After the anthropologist Franz Boas demonstrated a century ago that the children of poor European immigrants huddled in the slums of New York did not inherit the small head circumferences of their parents, many scientists gave up the popular assumption that these immigrants possessed tainted genes and began to study the environmental causes of this anatomical feature. The discovery that the virus that can cause cancer of the cervix may also be responsible for the sharp rise in cancers of the mouth, tongue, and throat in adults under age fifty, probably due to the increased frequency of oral sex, is likely to shift some inquiry from the malevolent consequences of smoking to the potential dangers of this sexual practice.

The investigators interested in temperament also have a more profitable set of questions to pursue. First, they have learned to appreciate the extreme specificity in nature. For example, it is important to distinguish between the site in the amygdala responsible for the observable signs of a temperamental bias, such as thrashing of limbs, crying, and arching of the back, and an adjacent site in the amygdala required to learn the events that trigger the neurons responsible for the former reactions. These two neuronal clusters are influenced by different molecules, receptors, and genes. This fact implies that some children might acquire a fear of large dogs following a single frightening experience, but lose the fear after several safe encounters. Others will require several fearful encounters before developing the phobia, but once the fear is established, find it difficult to suppress their fear and avoidance despite several years without an attack from a large dog. Because the prefrontal cortex exerts considerable control over the neuronal sites responsible for feelings, it is reasonable to assume that those who regularly experience the salient emotions of fear, revenge, or sexual arousal can learn to moderate the intensity of these feelings.

Epigenetics

A second set of questions is provoked by the recent discovery that environmental events, such as a prolonged famine, can add or remove a molecule from one of the bases within a gene and, as a result, influence the level of expression of that gene without changing the sequence of the four nucleotides that constitute the gene, like adding an accent mark above the letter *e* in the word "cliché." Identical twins who were separated at birth and raised in different homes had different patterns of gene expression caused by the addition or removal of these molecules. An experiential basis for alteration in a gene's activity is analogous to the acquired differences between carpenters and bank clerks in the thickness of the skin on the hands. Although the changes in genes created by a stressful event can be reversed, a small proportion is inherited by the next generation in a phenomenon called epigenetic inheritance. These observations will motivate investigators to discover how extensive this process is in humans and the specific experiences that have the power to alter or to reverse the change in the nucleotide.

Look for Patterns

A third group of questions originates in the recognition that individuals vary in patterns of features, rather than in single traits. Adolescent boys who had been low-reactive infants combine extreme sociability, low levels of anxiety to challenge, a low heart rate, and greater cortical activity in the left than in the right frontal lobe. An adolescent who possesses only one of these features should not automatically be classified as low-reactive. However, some investigators continue to rely on only one feature when they classify a person as anxious. For example, many scientists attribute anxiety to those who show a very large eyeblink reflex to a sudden loud sound while they are watching pictures with unpleasant content (bloodied soldiers or poisonous snakes). But every behavioral reaction and brain profile has more than one set of causal conditions. A large eyeblink reflex to a loud sound can occur if the person is thinking but is not anxious. Thus individuals who had large blink reflexes while looking at snakes might have been thinking about these animals when the loud sound occurred. Biologists typically use patterns of features when they assign an animal to a species category and are reluctant to rely on only one trait to distinguish among different breeds of cats or dogs.

The Gap between Brain and Mind

A final class of questions is provoked by the realization of a serious gap, or dissociation, between a measured brain state and a person's thought, feeling, or intended action. Past attempts to predict a psychological state or action from a brain profile at a high level of confidence have been unsuccessful, and for good reasons. First, the brain is a tightly interconnected set of structures affected by many molecules that influence each other in complex patterns of excitation and inhibition. Consider, as one example, the neurons located in a site that contributes to a person's preparation to approach or to avoid a desired event. Activity in this site is influenced by (1) neurons in the prefrontal cortex, amygdala, and brain stem, (2) the concentrations of at least six molecules that affect the excitability of these sites, (3) the concentrations of other molecules that control the duration of activity of the former substances, and (4) the density and availability of the relevant receptors. As a result, a particular level of activation in a restricted location in the brain could be the product of a large number of different mechanisms, and each could be the basis for a distinct psychological state.

There is a second reason why there cannot be a determinate relation between a brain profile produced by a particular event and a specific psychological outcome in a large number of individuals. Let us suppose that each distinct class of event produces a unique brain profile called "state E" (for event). State E is imposed on the person's usual brain state, which I shall call "state U" (for usual), which varies across people. The set of associations to the event, also unique across people, will create "state A" (for associations), which is imposed on the combination of states E and U. Although identical twins watching video clips designed to evoke sadness agreed that they felt sad, the members of the same twin pair had different brain profiles.

The brain state that scientists measure is a combination of states E, U, and A, which I shall call "brain state "F" (for final). Even if it were possible to measure this state in one hundred people, each state F profile would be the result of different combinations of states U and A, which varied across the one hundred individuals. Therefore it will be difficult, if not impossible, to predict with great accuracy the thoughts, feelings, or behaviors that might accompany the state F profiles produced by the incentive event. Free will is resting comfortably in the middle of this unpredictability!

A final frustration is the fact that the local context determines the specific action that is likely to follow state F. Scientists and everyone else want to know what people will do in the real world, rather than their reaction while lying perfectly still in the narrow tube of a magnetic scanner. Suppose that the event is the sight of a $100 bill lying on the ground. A person's reaction to the money will vary depending on whether he is alone in a parking garage, at a dinner party with friends, or saw a stranger a few feet ahead of him accidentally drop the bill from her coat. It should be obvious that it will be difficult to predict at a high level of confidence the psychological reactions of one hundred people to this particular event from measurements of their brain while lying in scanner when asked what they might do in this situation.

Even when the psychological state was restricted to the simple judgment of whether a warm stimulus applied to the hand felt pleasant or a cold stimulus felt unpleasant, the relation between the psychological judgment and the brain was not perfect. The person's judgment of pleasant or unpleasant agreed with the blood flow pattern to neurons that mediate pleasant or unpleasant feelings about 71 percent of the time. The level of agreement was much poorer when the warm and cold stimuli were applied simultaneously.

Many young adults who wish to be scientists are willing to work for ten years or more for the pleasure that accompanies the reward of a desired position at a university, hospital, or industrial or government laboratory. However, the amount of blood flow to a site that mediates the pleasure of a reward decreased when the delay between being told that a monetary reward was about to be delivered and receipt of the reward changed by only 9.5 seconds, from 4 to 13.5 seconds! If we assume that the blood flow evidence reveals a profound insight about the human ability to postpone gratification, it is impossible to understand the perseverance of young scientists over intervals of years. Thus there is a serious difference between the meaning of reward or pleasure based on evidence from brain functioning compared with the meaning inferred from the behaviors and feelings of humans in their natural settings. It is useful to remember that many of the wisest commentators on human nature have written that the joy is in the journey, not in the receipt of the goal being pursued.

The problem with too many conclusions in psychology, psychiatry, and neuroscience is that investigators are tempted to attribute a single meaning to a measure of brain or behavior that could have been caused by more than one condition and, therefore, assume different meanings. A state of fatigue can have many origins, and one has to know whether it was accompanied by a sore throat, fever, and evidence of a virus to arrive at the correct meaning of the fatigue. Similarly, increased activity in the amygdala, as measured by blood flow, could accompany uncertainty over delivery of an electric shock, the unexpected appearance of an erotic photograph, or brief exposure to a circle on a white background containing two black dots, and is often greater in individuals with very low heart rates who may not experience any strong emotion.

It is worth noting that when natural scientists discover a relation between two events—B is followed by A—they usually try to discover all the conditions that could have produced B. When one team of geneticists found that bombarding fruit flies with X-rays produced changes in anatomy that had to be due to genetic mutations, other biologists did not stop looking for other causes of mutations. Similarly, investigators continued to search for the conditions that lead to cardiac problems after investigators discovered that obesity was one risk factor. It has proven so difficult to find robust relations among an incentive, a feature of brain, and a behavioral outcome that scientists lucky enough to detect one of these precious secrets are understandably reluctant to search for other conditions that might produce the same outcome. Subsequent research might dilute the theoretical significance of the original discovery. This strategy of protecting a favored inference from refutation hinders progress in science. If we are to gain a satisfying understanding of the relations among experience, brain, and mind we must try to detect the flaws in an initial interpretation of an observation by ferreting out all the patterns of events and brain profiles that can create a particular psychological outcome.

The Need for a New Vocabulary

The new facts imply that neuroscientists must invent a special vocabulary for brain patterns and refrain from borrowing the psychologists' terms for emotions, actions, and thoughts. For example, many scientists call the brain pattern recorded while adults are looking at snakes "fear" and the pattern accompanying pictures of dirty toilets "disgust." However, fear and disgust are appropriate names only for human psychological states; they are inappropriate labels for brain states. By contrast, when clusters of neurons in different places discharge at the same frequency, neuroscientists say that the clusters are displaying "coherence." This feature of brains does not apply to people. Only humans can experience disgust; only neuronal clusters can be coherent.

The late Thomas Kuhn invented a nice example that makes this point clear. The French word *doux* is used to refer to the taste of honey, a soft touch, and bland-tasting soup. The English word "sweet" refers to the taste of honey and a soft touch as well, but it also names a victory on the athletic field and the middle strings of a tennis racquet, and it is never used to name bland-tasting soup. Thus, *doux* and "sweet" are not exact synonyms. Analogously, the word "fear" has different meanings when it refers to the brain profile evoked by pictures of snakes and when it refers to a person's declaration that she feels fearful when she sees a snake.

The challenge for the next generation of neuroscientists is to find a set of biological words that describe the varied patterns of brain activity produced by particular incentives. I rephrase an idea attributed to Thomas Huxley, Darwin's friend and fierce advocate for biological evolution, to convey the point of this discussion. The beautiful hope held by previous generations of neuroscientists that one day they would be able to translate psychological descriptions of thoughts, images, feelings, and intentions into sentences containing only words for neurons, molecules, and their physical and chemical properties has been destroyed by a collection of ugly facts.

Psychological states and the actions that follow emerge at the end of a cascade of processes that originated in the activation of select brain structures. But structures rarely reveal their ultimate functions. No naive observer examining a brain could guess its possible functions. One reason for the disguised quality of the functions that emerge from neuronal clusters is that the former always require more than the relevant structure in order to be actualized. For example, the primary functions of the ovum are to be fertilized and develop into an embryo. But that outcome requires a sperm and a very particular chemical environment in the vagina and uterus. The primary function of the muscles of the human heart is to deliver oxygen-rich blood to the body. But that function cannot be actualized without blood cells containing hemoglobin and a closed set of vessels that carry the blood to its targets and return it to the heart. Every thought, feeling, and action require activity in more than one brain site as well as a context that selects a particular thought, feeling, or action. These are some of the reasons why we remain unable to understand how any psychological phenomenon could emerge from certain clusters of activated neurons.

All of these questions were less well articulated when Chess and Thomas first suggested their nine temperamental biases. The fact that these queries can be stated succinctly is testimony to the extraordinary progress of the past fifty years. An old Swedish proverb captures the gifts that time has bestowed on so many hardworking scientists: "The afternoon knows what the morning never suspected."

Coda

The lively interest in human temperaments is motivating more-extensive study of the feelings and emotions that are harder to measure than behavior. Emotions are analogous to the hidden molecular structures responsible for the appearances of plants and animals that could not be quantified until new technologies were invented. Future research will alert psychiatrists, psychologists, and the public to the importance of a person's private feelings. At the moment, we do not possess procedures sensitive enough to measure with great accuracy either the quality of various conscious feelings or the brain states that are their foundation. However, future investigators should be better able to detect these elusive states and their foundations in brain activity. These victories will provide a deeper understanding of the reasons for the differences among humans in their emotional patinas and their vulnerability to the disturbing symptoms of chronic anxiety, depression, addiction, callousness, and cognitive impairments that continue to plague our species.

Glossary

acetylcholine. A neurotransmitter active in both the brain and the autonomic nervous system. It is especially important in the frontal lobe functions of attention and learning.

adenine. One of the four nucleotides in the DNA molecule.

allele. A different form of a gene created by a change in DNA sequence at a specific location on the gene.

amino acids. Molecules that combine to form proteins.

amygdala. A small, almond-shaped set of neurons located near the temporal lobe. It receives information from all sensory sources, influences many bodily reactions, and contributes to many emotions.

anorexia nervosa. An eating disorder in which individuals severely restrict eating. It most often affects adolescent females.

anterior cingulate cortex (ACC). A part of the cingulate cortex near the frontal lobe that is involved in autonomic and cognitive functions, and the modulation of emotion.

attention-deficit/hyperactivity disorder (ADHD). A mental disorder characterized by hyperactivity, or difficulty maintaining attention, or both, that interferes with the ability to meet the requirements of an academic setting. ADHD is the most common disorder of children, affecting 3 to 5 percent of seven- to eight-year-olds.

autism. A family of serious disorders characterized by a core set of symptoms with different causes. The major symptoms are inappropriate social behavior, seriously retarded language development, inappropriate affect, and repetitions of motor responses, such as banging of the head and picking of the skin, without any obvious provocation.

autoimmune disease. An abnormal immune reaction in which the immune system attacks its own cells, causing diseases such as multiple sclerosis, Addison's disease, and rheumatoid arthritis.

biologically prepared. Having biological characteristics that confer a special receptivity to particular events or a special ease of displaying particular responses that are specific to a species.

blood flow. Changes in the amount of blood arriving at specific locations in the brain, measured in a magnetic scanner.

bulimia. An eating disorder characterized by repeated binge eating followed by self-induced vomiting or purging.

CAT scan. A non-invasive medical test using a combination of special X-ray equipment and computers to produce multiple images of the inside of the body.

clone. A group of identical cells derived from a common mother cell and having the same genes as the mother cell.

conduct disorder. A pattern of asocial behavior in children or adolescents characterized by verbal and physical aggression, unusually cruel behavior toward people or animals, truancy, and/or the performance of criminal actions such as vandalism and stealing.

congenital adrenal hyperplasia (CAH). A family of diseases caused by mutations in the genes important in the production of cortisol and sex hormones by the adrenal glands. Conditions associated with CAH include ambiguous genitals, precocious puberty, masculine features, or irregular menstrual cycles.

cortisol. A hormone produced by the adrenal cortex in response to stress that causes increased blood pressure, the release of blood sugar, and abnormal activity of the immune system.

cytokine. Any one of a number of molecular substances secreted by the immune system that carry signals between cells.

cytosine. One of the four nucleotides in a DNA molecule.

Diagnostic and Statistic Manual of Mental Disorders (DSM). The guide for diagnosis that psychiatrists use when deciding on the mental illness category to which a person belongs.

DNA. The elementary molecular component of a gene, comprising repetitions of pairs of four molecules called bases, with the names adenine, guanine, cytosine, and thymine.

dopamine. A neurotransmitter involved in voluntary movement, motivation, reward, sleep, mood, attention, and learning.

epigenetics. Changes in the chemical structure of a gene, other than a rearrangement in the order of the nucleotides, caused by events in the environment or changes in the body. Some epigenetic changes are inherited.

estrogen. A group of steroid molecules that are the primary female sex hormones, including estradiol, estrone, and estriol.

frontal lobe. One of the four divisions of each cerebral hemisphere, lying directly behind the forehead. It contains many dopamine-sensitive neurons and is involved in executive functions, including predicting future consequences of current actions, choosing between good and bad, moderating social behavior, and maintaining information in working memory.

gene. The basic unit of heredity, usually defined as a locatable region of a DNA sequence.

guanine. One of the four nucleotides in the DNA molecule.

hallucinations. The experience of a sound, sight, smell, or touch, in the absence of any external stimulus, that is vivid and appears to be real. Hallucinations are most often present as a symptom of schizophrenia.

high-reactive. A term referring to four-month-old infants who display high levels of motor activity and crying in response to unfamiliar stimuli.

honne. The frame of mind of a Japanese adult who is prepared to express his or her beliefs and emotions sincerely when interacting with an intimate.

hypothalamus. A small cluster of neurons that link the brain to the endocrine system via the pituitary gland.

identification. The psychological state created by a combination of the belief that a person shares important features with another person or group and the experience of vicarious emotion appropriate to the person or group with whom the individual is identified.

inferior colliculus. A small neural structure in the midbrain that receives sound stimulation from the ear and transmits it to the auditory cortex by way of the thalamus.

insula. A brain structure located between the temporal and parietal lobes that is involved in awareness of body activity and emotion.

intron. A string of DNA in the nucleus that is deleted before a copy is transported to the cell to make amino acids.

low-reactive. A term referring to four-month-old infants who display minimal motor activity and crying in response to unfamiliar events.

MAO. The abbreviation for monoamine oxidase, a family of enzymes that reduce the concentration of a group of molecules called monoamines, including dopamine, serotonin, and norepinephrine.

melatonin. A naturally occurring hormone important in the regulation of circadian rhythms. In pregnancy, maternal melatonin influences the genes, antioxidant activity, and synthesis of particular molecules in the embryo.

multiple personality disorder (dissociative identity disorder). A condition in which a person displays distinctly different personalities. Some psychiatrists question the validity of multiple personality as a diagnosis.

multiple sclerosis. An autoimmune disease affecting the brain and spinal cord, causing a loss of balance and problems with movement of the arms and legs.

neural crest. A transient set of cells in the young embryo that give rise to the autonomic nervous system, facial bone, sensory ganglia, and the cells that make melanin.

norepinephrine. A neurotransmitter affecting many parts of the brain involved in attention, action, heart rate, and blood flow.

nucleus accumbens. A collection of neurons that plays an important role in reward systems and feelings of pleasure.

obsessive-compulsive disorder (OCD). A mental disorder characterized by intrusive thoughts, repetitive compulsive behaviors, or combinations of thoughts and compulsions. Examples include repetitive washing of the hands, hoarding paper clips, and an excessive preoccupation with sexual, religious, or aggressive ideas.

opioids. A family of molecules found principally in the central nervous system and the gastrointestinal tract that reduce the perception of pain.

orbitofrontal cortex (OFC). A region of the frontal lobe that integrates information from the thalamus, amygdala, insula, and other parts of the brain.

oxytocin. A hormone that acts as a neurotransmitter. It is released in large amounts during labor, nursing, and sexual behavior.

panic disorder. Sudden fear or anxiety caused by unexpected increases in heart rate, blood pressure, respiration, and other bodily processes, such as dizziness, that appear to have no obvious trigger. Panic attacks can last less than a minute or as long as twenty minutes. Individuals who are overly frightened of such experiences become reluctant to leave the familiar home setting and are called agoraphobic.

parasympathetic nervous system. The division of the autonomic nervous system that is complementary to the sympathetic nervous system and involved in the activities of rest and digestion.

parietal lobe. A large area of cortex in the posterior part of the brain where sensory information is integrated, allowing animals and humans to navigate and locate objects in space.

Parkinson's disease. A disorder characterized by muscle rigidity, tremor of the hands, and slow movement caused primarily by insufficient secretion of dopamine.

phobic disorder. An irrational fear accompanied by a conscious avoidance of the feared object. The three major types are social phobia, specific phobias of animals or heights, and agoraphobia.

post-traumatic stress disorder (PTSD). An anxiety disorder that develops after a person has been exposed to a traumatic event, such as witnessing someone's death, a threat to the person's life, or a violent sexual attack.

prefrontal cortex. The front part of the cerebral cortex, involved in planning, decision making, working memory, and the orchestration of thoughts, feelings, and actions.

proteins. Complex molecular structures composed of amino acids.

receptor. A protein, usually embedded in the membrane of a cell, to which a particular molecule attaches. When the molecule binds to the receptor, the latter undergoes a change in conformation that initiates a response from the cell.

sensory threshold. A theoretical idea referring to the lowest intensity that a person can detect.

serotonin transporter. A protein that transports the molecule serotonin from the synaptic space into a presynaptic neuron, reducing the concentration of serotonin in the synapse.

social anxiety. The experience of discomfort, fear, or worry when one anticipates or is involved in social interaction with others.

social class. The relative rank of an individual or family determined by the qualities that a society regards as desirable. In contemporary Western societies, wealth, education, and vocation are the usual symbols of class.

stereotypes. A relatively inflexible, abstract semantic category for a group of people, usually ethnic, religious, and national categories.

sympathetic nervous system. A branch of the autonomic nervous system with neurons that lie in a chain along the spinal cord. It becomes active during times of stress and mediates changes in heart rate, blood pressure, circulatory vessels, muscles, stomach, and reproductive organs.

tatemae. The frame of mind of a Japanese adult interacting with a non-intimate in a conventional setting, which requires a less forthright manner.

temperament. The initial biases in infants and young children for certain feelings and behaviors due to inherited differences in anatomy or physiology or to prenatal events.

testosterone. A steroid hormone secreted by the male testes and in much smaller amounts by the ovaries and adrenal glands. Testosterone is the principle male sex hormone and influences the establishment of the male sex organs as well as the changes that occur at puberty.

2D:4D. The ratio of the lengths of the index to the ring finger, determined during the prenatal months by the amount of testosterone secreted by the male fetus. Most males have a smaller ratio than females.

vasopressin. A hormone important in the body's retention of water. It is also released during sexual behavior and is more active in males than in females.

ventral tegmentum. A group of neurons in the midbrain that secretes dopamine and sends this molecule to many parts of the brain.

ventromedial prefrontal cortex. A part of the prefrontal cortex that lies between the two hemispheres and is involved in the regulation of emotions and decision making.

Y-antigen. A protein secreted by the Y chromosome that is responsible for the primary sex determination in the male.

Selected Bibliography

Chapter 1

Brummett, B. H., S. H. Boyle, I. C. Siegler, C. M. Kuhn, A. Ashley-Koch, C. R. Jonassaint, S. Zuchner, A. Collins, and R. B. Williams. "Effects of Environmental Stress and Gender on Associations among Symptoms of Depression and the Serotonin Transporter Gene Linked Polymorphic (5-HTTPLR)." *Behavior Genetics* 38 (2008): 34–43.

Chess, S., and A. Thomas. "Genesis and Evolution of Behavior Disorders." *American Journal of Psychiatry* 141 (1984): 1–9.

Gortmaker, S. L., J. Kagan, A. Caspi, and P. A. Silva. "Daylight during Pregnancy and Shyness in Children." *Developmental Psychobiology* 31 (1997): 107–114.

Jay, T. "The Utility and Ubiquity of Taboo Words." *Perspectives on Psychological Science* 4 (2009): 153–161.

Kagan, J. *Birth to Maturity*. New York: John Wiley, 1962.

———. *Galen's Prophecy*. New York: Basic Books, 1994.

Kagan, J., R. Kearsley, and P. Zelazo. *Infancy*. Cambridge, MA: Harvard University Press, 1978.

Kagan, J., and N. Snidman. *The Long Shadow of Temperament*. Cambridge, MA: Harvard University Press, 2004.

Kagan, J., N. Snidman, V. Kahn, and S. Towsley. "The Preservation of Two Infant Temperaments into Adolescence." *Monographs of the Society for Research in Child Development* 72 (2007): 1–75.

Karere, G. M., E. L. Kinnally, J. N. Sanchez, T. R. Famula, L. A. Lyons, and J. P. Capitanio. "What Is an Adverse Environment?" *Biological Psychiatry*. In press.

King. S., A. Mancini-Marie, A. Brunet, E. Walker, M. J. Meaney, and D. P. Laplante. "Prenatal Maternal Stress from a Natural Disaster Predicts Dermatoglyphic Asymmetry in Humans." *Development and Psychopathology* 21 (2009): 343–353.

Koenen, K. C., A. B. Amstadter, K. J. Ruggiero, R. Acierno, S. Galea, D. G. Kilpatrick, and J. Gelerntner. "RGS2 and Generalized Anxiety Disorder in an Epidemiological Sample of Hurricane-Exposed Adults." *Depression and Anxiety* 26 (2009): 309–315.

Patterson, P. H. "Pregnancy, Immunity, Schizophrenia, and Autism." *Engineering and Science* 3 (2006): 11–21.

Pharoah, P. O. D., S. V. Glinianaia, and J. Rankin. "Congenital Anomalies in Multiple Births after Loss of a Conceptus." *Human Reproduction* 24 (2009): 726–731.

Willer, C. J., D. A. Dyment, A. D. Sadovnick, P. M. Rothwell, T. J. Murray, and G. C. Ebers. "Timing of Birth and Risk of Multiple Sclerosis." *British Medical Journal* 330 (2005): 120–125.

Woolf, Virginia. "Craftsmanship," from the 1937 radio series "Words Fail Me." *The Death of the Moth and other essays* (1942). http://ebooks.adelaide. edu.au/w/woolf/virginia/w91d/

Chapter 2

Buhr, K., and M. J. Dugas. "The Intolerance of Uncertainty Scale." *Behaviour Research and Therapy* 40 (2002): 931–945.

Feng, X., D. S. Shaw, and J. S. Silk. "Developmental Trajectories of Anxiety Symptoms among Boys across Early and Middle Childhood." *Journal of Abnormal Psychology* 117 (2008): 32–47.

Fox, N. A., H. A. Henderson, K. H. Rubin, S. D. Calkins, and L. A. Schmidt. "Continuity and Discontinuity of Behavioral Inhibition and Exuberance." *Child Development* 72 (2001): 1–21.

Fox, N. A., K. H. Rubin, S. D. Calkins, T. R. Marshall, R. J. Coplan, and S. W. Porges. "Frontal Activation Asymmetry and Social Competence at Four Years of Age." *Child Development* 66 (1995): 1770–1784.

Hebb, D. O. "On the Nature of Fear." *Psychological Review* 53 (1946): 259–276.

Henderson, M., and M. Hotopf. "Childhood Temperament and Long-Term Sickness Absence in Adult Life." *British Journal of Psychiatry* 194 (2009): 220–223.

Koenigs, M., E. D. Huey, M. Calamia, V. Raymont, D. Tranel, and J. Grafman. "Distinct Regions of Prefrontal Cortex Mediate Resistance and Vulnerability to Depression." *Journal of Neuroscience* 28 (2008): 12331–12348.

Kong, J., T. J. Kaptchuk, G. Polich, I. Kirsch, M. Vangel, C. Zylmen, B. Rosen, and R. Gollub. "Expectancy and Treatment Interaction." *Neuroimage* 45 (2009): 940–949.

Luk, C. H., and J. D. Wallis. "Dynamic Encoding of Responses and Outcomes by Neurons in Medial Prefrontal Cortex." *Journal of Neuroscience* 29 (2009): 7526–7539.

Mojtabai, R. "Parental Psychopathology and Childhood Atopic Disorders in the Community." *Psychosomatic Medicine* 67 (2005): 448–453.

Moskovitz, S. *Love Despite Hate*. New York: Schocken Books, 1982.

Robinson, J. L., J. Kagan, J. S. Reznick, and R. Corley. "The Heritability of Inhibited and Uninhibited Behavior: A Twin Study." *Developmental Psychology* 28 (1992): 1030–1037.

Rothbart, M. K., and J. E. Bates. "Temperament." In N. Eisenberg, ed., *Social, Emotional, and Personality Development*, 99–166. Vol. 3 of *Handbook of Child Psychology*, edited by W. Damon and R. M. Lerner. 6th ed. New York: John Wiley, 2006.

Rubin, K. H., K. D. Burgess, and D. D. Hastings. "Stability and Social Behavioral Consequences of Toddlers' Inhibited Temperament and Parenting Behaviors." *Child Development* 73 (2002): 483–495.

Schwartz, C. E., P. S. Kunwar, D. N, Greve, L. R. Moran, et al. "Structural Differences in Adult Orbital and Ventromedial Prefrontal Cortex Predicted by Infant Temperament at 4 Months of Age." *Archives of General Psychiatry* 67 (2010): 1-7.

Zhou, X., G. Saucier, G. Dingguo, and J. Liu. "The Factor Structure of Chinese Personality Terms." *Journal of Personality* 77 (2009): 363–400.

Chapter 3

Abel, E. L., and M. L. Kruger. "Performance of Older versus Younger Brothers." *Perceptual and Motor Skills* 105 (2007): 1117–1118.

Cockerham, W. C. *Social Causes of Health and Disease* (London: Polity Press).

Firkowska, A., A. Ostrowska, M. Sokolowska, Z. Stein, M. Susser, and I. Wald. "Cognitive Development and Social Policy." *Science* 200 (1978): 1357–1362.

Koch, H. L. "Some Emotional Attitudes of a Young Child in Relation to Characteristics of His Siblings." *Child Development* 27 (1956): 393–426.

Lau, C. "Child Prostitution in Thailand." *Journal of Child Health Care* 12 (2008):145–156.

Mobbs, D. R., M. Meyer Yu, L. Passamonti, B. Seymour, A. J. Calder, S. Schweizer, C. D. Frith, and T. Dalgeish. "A Key Role for Similarity in Vicarious Reward." *Science* 324 (2009): 900.

Robisheaux, T. *The Last Witch of Langenburg*. New York: W. W. Norton, 2009.

Simm, R. W., and L. E. Nath. "Gender and Emotion." *American Journal of Sociology* 109 (2004): 1137–1176.

Sulloway, F. J. *Born to Rebel*. New York: Random House, 1996.

Chapter 4

Brody, L. *Gender, Emotion, and the Family*. Cambridge, MA: Harvard University Press, 1999.

Carter, C. S. "Developmental Consequences of Oxytocin." *Physiology and Behavior* 79 (2003): 383–397.

Coates, J. N., M. Gurnell, and A. Rustichini. "Second-to-Fourth Digit Ratio Predicts Success among High-Frequency Financial Traders." *Proceedings of the National Academy of Sciences* 106 (2009): 623–628.

Federman, D. D. "The Biology of Human Sex Differences." *New England Journal of Medicine* 354 (2006): 1507–1514.

Hassett, J. M., E. R. Siebert, and K. Wallen. "Sex Differences in Rhesus Monkey Toy Preferences Parallel Those of Children." *Hormones and Behavior* 54 (2008): 359–364.

Karelina, K., and G. J. Norman. "Oxytocin Influence on the Nucleus of the Solitary Tract." *Journal of Neuroscience* 29 (2009): 4689–4687.

King, J. E., A. Weiss, and M. M. Sisco. "Aping Humans: Age and Sex Effects in Chimpanzee (Pan troglodytes) and Human (Homo sapiens) Personality." *Journal of Comparative Psychology* (2009): 1–10.

Koscik, T., D. O'Leary, D. J. Moser, N. C. Andreasen, and P. Nopoulos. "Sex Differences in Parietal Lobe Morphology." *Brain and Cognition* 69 (2009): 451–459.

Leknes, S., and I. Tracey. "A Common Neurobiology for Pain and Pleasure." *Nature Reviews: Neuroscience* 9 (2008): 314–320.

Mathews, G. A., B. A. Fane, G. S. Conway, C. G. D. Brook, and M. Hines. "Personality and Congenital Adrenal Hyperplasia." *Hormones and Behavior* 55 (2009): 285–291.

Meyer, G., J. Schwertfeger, M. S. Exton, O. E. Janssen, W. Knapp, M. A. Stadler, M. Schedlowski, and T. H. C. Kruger. "Neuroendocrine Response to Casino Gambling in Problem Gamblers." *Psychoneuroendocrinology* 29 (2004):1272–1280.

Munro, A., M. E. McCaul, D. F. Wong, L. M. Oswald, Y. Zhou, J. Brasic, H. Kuwabara, A. Kumar, M. Alexander, W. Ye, and G. S. Wand. "Sex Differences in Striatal Dopamine Release in Healthy Adults." *Biological Psychiatry* 59 (2006): 966–974.

Neufang, S., K. Specht, M. Hausmann, O. Gunturkun, B. Herpertz-Dahlmann, G. R. Fink, and K. Conrad. "Sex Differences and the Impact of Steroid Hormones on the Developing Human Brain." *Cerebral Cortex* 19 (2009): 464–473.

Ross, H. E., S. M. Freeman;, L. L. Spiegel, X. Ren, E. F. Terwilliger, and L. J. Young. "Variation in Oxytocin Receptor Density in the Nucleus Accumbens Has Differential Effects on Affiliative Behaviors in Monogamous and Polygamous Voles." *Journal of Neuroscience* 29 (2009): 1312–1318.

von Stumm, S., T. Chammoro-Premuzic, and A. Furnham. "Decomposing Self-Estimates of Intelligence." *British Journal of Psychology* 100 (2009): 429–442.

Wallen, M. S., K. J. Zucker, T. D. Steensma, and P. T. Cohen-Kettenis. "2D:4D Finger-Length Ratios in Children and Adults with Gender Identity Disorder." *Hormones and Behavior* 54 (2008): 450–454.

Whiting, B. B., and J. W. M. Whiting. *Children of Six Cultures: A Psycho-Cultural Analysis.* Cambridge, MA: Harvard University Press, 1975.

Chapter 5

Anderson, D. J. "Molecular Control of Cell Fate in the Neural Crest." *Annual Review of Neuroscience* 16 (1993): 129–158.

Barnes, B., and J. Dupre. *Genomes and What to Make of Them.* Chicago: University of Chicago Press, 2008.

Cavalli-Sforza, L. L., and F. Cavalli-Sforza. *The Great Human Diasporas.* Reading, MA: Addison-Wesley, 1995.

Chua, H. F., J. E. Boland, and R. E. Nisbett. "Cultural Variation in Eye Movements during Scene Perception." *Proceedings of the National Academy of Sciences* 102 (2005): 12629–12633.

Goldstein, D. B. *Jacob's Legacy.* New Haven, CT: Yale University Press, 2008.

Grant, R., and B. R. Grant. *How and Why Species Multiply.* Princeton, NJ: Princeton University Press, 2008.

Kim, H. S., D. K. Sherman, and S. E. Taylor. "Culture and Social Support." *American Psychologist* 63 (2008): 518–526.

Kirschner, M. W., and J. C. Gerhart. *The Plausibility of Life.* New Haven, CT: Yale University Press, 2005.

Le, T. T., L. G. Farkas, R. C. K. Ngim, L. S. Levin, and C. R. Forrest. "Proportionality in Asian and North American Caucasian Faces Using Neoclassical Facial Canons as Criteria." *Aesthetic Plastic Surgery* 26 (2002): 64–69.

Li, J. Z., D. M. Absher, H. Tang, A. M. Southwick, A. M. Casto, S. Ramachandran, H. M. Cann, G. S. Barsh, M. Feldman, L. L. Cavalli-Sforza, and R. M. Myers. "World-Wide Human Relationships Inferred from Genome-Wide Patterns of Variation." *Science* 319 (2008): 1100–1104.

Masuda, T., R. Gonzalez, L. Kwan, and R. E. Nisbett. "Culture and Aesthetic Preference: Comparing the Attention to Context of East Asians and Americans." *Personality and Social Psychology Bulletin* 34 (2008): 1260–1275.

Trut, L. N. "Early Canid Domestication." *American Scientist* 87 (1999): 160–169.

Chapter 6

al-Mujawir, I. *A Traveler in Thirteenth Century Arabia*. London: Hakluyt Society, 2008.

Baatz, S. *For the Thrill of It*. New York: HarperCollins, 2008.

Blom, P. *The Vertigo Years*. New York: Perseus Books, 2008.

Cass, L. K., and C. B. Thomas. *Childhood Pathology and Later Adjustment*. New York: John Wiley, 1979.

Clarvit, S. R., F. R. Schneier, and M. R. Leibowitz. "The Offensive Subtype of Taijin-Kyofu-Sho in New York City." *Journal of Clinical Psychiatry* 57 (1996): 523–527.

Flynn, K. A. "In Their Own Voices: Women Who Were Sexually Abused by Members of the Clergy." *Journal of Child Sex Abuse* 17 (2008): 216–237.

Himle, J. A., R. E. Baser, R. J. Taylor, R. D. Campbell, and J. S. Jackson. "Anxiety Disorders among African Americans, Blacks of Caribbean Descent, and Non-Hispanic Whites in the United States." *Journal of Anxiety Disorders* 23 (2009): 578–590.

Koutsouleris, N., E. M. Meisenzahl, C. Davatzikos, R. Bottlender, T. Frodl, J. Scheuerecker, G. Schmitt, T. Zetzsche, P. Decker, M. Reiser, H. J. Moller, and C. Gaser. "Use of Neuroanatomical Pattern Classification to Identify Subjects in At-Risk Mental States of Psychosis and Predict Disease Transition." *Archives of General Psychiatry* 66 (2009): 700–712.

Levine, S. Z., and J. Rabinowitz. "A Population-Based Examination of the Role of Years of Education, Age of Onset, and Sex on the Consequences of Schizophrenia." *Psychiatry Research* 168: 14–17.

McHugh, P. R. *Try to Remember.* Washington, D.C.: Dana Press, 2008.

Merikangas, K. R., and N. Risch. "Will the Genomic Revolution Revolutionize Psychiatry?" *American Journal of Psychiatry* 160 (2003): 625–635.

Moisin, L. *Kid Rex.* Toronto: E. C. W. Press, 2008.

Nydegger, R. *Understanding and Treating Depression.* Westport, CT: Praeger, 2008.

Seedat, S., K. M. Scott, M. C. Angermeyer, P. Bergland, E. J. Bromet, T. S. Brugha, K. Demyttenaere, et al. "Cross-National Associations between Gender and Mental Health Disorders in the World Health Organization World Mental Health Surveys." *Archives of General Psychiatry* 66 (2009): 785–795.

Sereny, G. *Cries Unheard.* New York: Henry Holt, 1998.

Smoller, J. W., E. Gardner-Schuster, and M. Misiaszek. "Genetics of Anxiety." *Depression and Anxiety* 25 (2008): 368–377.

Strause, J. *Alice James.* Boston: Houghton Mifflin, 1980.

Tsapakis, E. M., F. Soldani, L. Tondo, and R. J. Baldessarini. "Efficacy of Antidepressants in Juvenile Depression: Meta-analysis." *British Journal of Psychiatry* 193 (2008): 10–17.

Warner, V., P. Wickramaratne, and M. M. Weisman. "The Role of Fear and Anxiety in the Familial Risk for Major Depression: A Three-Generation Study." *Psychological Medicine* 38 (2008): 1543–1556.

Wentz, E., I. C. Gillberg, H. Anckarsater, C. Gillberg, and M. Rastam. "Adolescent-onset anorexia nervosa: 18-year outcome." *British Journal of Psychiatry* 194 (2009): 168–174.

Wilhelm, F. H., and W. T. Roth. "The Somatic Symptom Paradox in DSM-IV Anxiety Disorders." *Biological Psychology* 57 (2001): 105–140.

Chapter 7

Adler, N. E., T. Boyce, M. A. Chesney, S. Cohen, S. Folkman, R. L. Kahn, and S. L. Syme. "Socio-economic Status and Health." *American Psychologist* 49 (1994): 15–24.

Gregorios-Pippas, L., P. N. Tobler, and W. Schultz. "Short-Term Temporal Discounting of Reward Value in Human Ventral Striatum." *Journal of Neurophysiology* 101 (2009): 1507–1523.

Heaney, S. *Sweeney Astray*. New York: Farrar Straus Giroux, 1983.

Kochanska, G. "Socialization and Temperament in the Development of Guilt and Conscience." *Child Development* 62 (1991): 1379–1392.

Miller, G., E. Chen, and S. W. Cole. "Health Psychology: Developing Biologically Plausible Models Linking the Social World and Physical Health." *Annual Review of Psychology* 60 (2009): 1–24.

Rolls, E. T., F. Grabenhorst, and L. Franco. "Prediction of Subjective Affective State from Brain Activity." *Journal of Neurophysiology* 101 (2009): 1294–1308.

Sexton, A. *Love Poems*. Boston: Houghton Mifflin, 1967.

Spatz, C. S., K. DuMont, and S. J. Czaja. "A Prospective Investigation of Major Depressive Disorder and Comorbidity in Abused and Neglected Children Grown Up." *Archives of General Psychiatry* 64 (2007): 49–56.

Index

Other Dana Press Books

www.dana.org/news/danapressbooks

Books for General Readers

Brain and Mind

TREATING THE BRAIN: What the Best Doctors Know
Walter G. Bradley, DM, FRCP

Using patient case histories, *Treating the Brain* explains the causes, diagnosis, prognosis, and treatment of a wide range of frequently diagnosed disorders, including Alzheimer's, migraines, stroke, epilepsy, and Parkinson's.
9 illustrations.

Cloth • 336 pp • ISBN-13: 978-1-932594-46-1 • $25.00

DEEP BRAIN STIMULATION:
A New Treatment Shows Promise in the Most Difficult Cases
Jamie Talan

An award-winning science writer has penned the first general-audience book to explore the benefits and risks of this cutting-edge technology, which is producing promising results for a wide range of brain disorders.

Cloth• 200 pp • ISBN-13: 978-1-932594-37-9 • $25.00

TRY TO REMEMBER: Psychiatry's Clash Over Meaning, Memory, and Mind
Paul R. McHugh, M.D.

Prominent psychiatrist and author Paul McHugh chronicles his battle to put right what has gone wrong in psychiatry. McHugh takes on such controversial subjects as "recovered memories," multiple personalities, and the overdiagnosis of PTSD.

Cloth • 300 pp • ISBN-13: 978-1-932594-39-3 • $25.00

CEREBRUM 2010: Emerging Ideas in Brain Science
Foreword by Benjamin S. Carson Sr., M.D.

Cerebrum 2010 offers a feast for readers keen to know what the world's leading thinkers see as the newest ideas and implications arising from discoveries about the brain. Preeminent scientists present their research or argue their point of view about such topics as the teen brain, how arts education affects intelligence, and the limitations of brain imaging.

Paper • 252 pp • ISBN-13: 978-1-932594-49-2 • $14.95

CEREBRUM 2009: Emerging Ideas in Brain Science
Foreword by Thomas R. Insel, M.D.

Why does mental fuzziness follow heart surgery? Can brain scans predict how you'll vote? How life-threatening is hidden brain injury? Leading scientists and writers tackle these and other challenging issues.

Paper • 188 pp • ISBN-13: 978-1-932594-44-7 • $14.95

CEREBRUM 2008: Emerging Ideas in Brain Science

Foreword by Carl Zimmer

Is free will an illusion? Why must we remember the past to envision the future? How can architecture help Alzheimer's patients? This edition presents these and 10 other topics.

Paper • 225 pp • ISBN-13: 978-1-932594-33-1 • $14.95

CEREBRUM 2007: Emerging Ideas in Brain Science

Foreword by Bruce S. McEwen, Ph.D.

How dangerous is adult sleepwalking? Is happiness hard-wired? Could an elephant be the next Picasso? Prominent neuroscientists and other thinkers explore a year's worth of topics.

Paper • 243 pp • ISBN-13: 978-1-932594-24-9 • $14.95

Visit Cerebrum online at www.dana.org/news/cerebrum.

YOUR BRAIN ON CUBS: Inside the Heads of Players and Fans

Dan Gordon, Editor

Our brains light up with the rush that accompanies a come-from-behind win—and the crush of a disappointing loss. Brain research also offers new insight into how players become experts. Neuroscientists and science writers explore these topics and more in this intriguing look at talent and triumph on the field and our devotion in the stands.

6 illustrations.

Cloth • 150 pp • ISBN-13: 978-1-932594-28-7 • $19.95

THE NEUROSCIENCE OF FAIR PLAY:
Why We (Usually) Follow the Golden Rule

Donald W. Pfaff, Ph.D.

A distinguished neuroscientist presents a rock-solid hypothesis of why humans across time and geography have such similar notions of good and bad, right and wrong.

10 illustrations.

Cloth • 234 pp • ISBN-13: 978-1-932594-27-0 • $20.95

BEST OF THE BRAIN FROM SCIENTIFIC AMERICAN:
Mind, Matter, and Tomorrow's Brain

Floyd E. Bloom, M.D., Editor

Top neuroscientist Floyd E. Bloom has selected the most fascinating brain-related articles from *Scientific American* and *Scientific American Mind* since 1999 in this collection.

30 illustrations.

Cloth • 300 pp • ISBN-13: 978-1-932594-22-5 • $25.00

MIND WARS: Brain Research and National Defense

Jonathan D. Moreno, Ph.D.

A leading ethicist examines national security agencies' work on defense applications of brain science, and the ethical issues to consider.

Cloth • 210 pp • ISBN-10: 1-932594-16-7 • $23.95

THE DANA GUIDE TO BRAIN HEALTH:
A Practical Family Reference from Medical Experts (with CD-ROM)

Floyd E. Bloom, M.D., M. Flint Beal, M.D., and David J. Kupfer, M.D., Editors

Foreword by William Safire

A complete, authoritative, family-friendly guide to the brain's development, health, and disorders. 16 full-color pages and more than 200 black-and-white drawings.

Paper (with CD-ROM) • 733 pp • ISBN-10: 1-932594-10-8 • $25.00

THE CREATING BRAIN: The Neuroscience of Genius

Nancy C. Andreasen, M.D., Ph.D.

A noted psychiatrist and best-selling author explores how the brain achieves creative breakthroughs, including questions such as how creative people are different and the difference between genius and intelligence.

33 illustrations/photos.

Cloth • 197 pp • ISBN-10: 1-932594-07-8 • $23.95

THE ETHICAL BRAIN

Michael S. Gazzaniga, Ph.D.

Explores how the lessons of neuroscience help resolve today's ethical dilemmas, ranging from when life begins to free will and criminal responsibility.

Cloth • 201 pp • ISBN-10: 1-932594-01-9 • $25.00

A GOOD START IN LIFE:
Understanding Your Child's Brain and Behavior from Birth to Age 6

Norbert Herschkowitz, M.D., and Elinore Chapman Herschkowitz

The authors show how brain development shapes a child's personality and behavior, discussing appropriate rule-setting, the child's moral sense, temperament, language, playing, aggression, impulse control, and empathy.

13 illustrations.

Cloth • 283 pp • ISBN-10: 0-309-07639-0 • $22.95

Paper (Updated with new material) • 312 pp • ISBN-10: 0-9723830-5-0 • $13.95

BACK FROM THE BRINK:
How Crises Spur Doctors to New Discoveries about the Brain

Edward J. Sylvester

In two academic medical centers, Columbia's New York Presbyterian and Johns Hopkins Medical Institutions, a new breed of doctor, the neurointensivist, saves patients with life-threatening brain injuries.

16 illustrations/photos.

Cloth • 296 pp • ISBN-10: 0-9723830-4-2 • $25.00

THE BARD ON THE BRAIN:
Understanding the Mind Through the Art of Shakespeare and the Science of Brain Imaging

Paul M. Matthews, M.D., and Jeffrey McQuain, Ph.D. • *Foreword by Diane Ackerman*

Explores the beauty and mystery of the human mind and the workings of the brain, following the path the Bard pointed out in 35 of the most famous speeches from his plays.
100 illustrations.

Cloth • 248 pp • ISBN-10: 0-9723830-2-6 • $35.00

STRIKING BACK AT STROKE: A Doctor-Patient Journal

Cleo Hutton and Louis R. Caplan, M.D.

A personal account, with medical guidance from a leading neurologist, for anyone enduring the changes that a stroke can bring to a life, a family, and a sense of self.
15 illustrations.

Cloth • 240 pp • ISBN-10: 0-9723830-1-8 • $27.00

UNDERSTANDING DEPRESSION:
What We Know and What You Can Do About It

J. Raymond DePaulo, Jr., M.D., and Leslie Alan Horvitz

Foreword by Kay Redfield Jamison, Ph.D.

What depression is, who gets it and why, what happens in the brain, troubles that come with the illness, and the treatments that work.

Cloth • 304 pp • ISBN-10: 0-471-39552-8 • $24.95
Paper • 296 pp • ISBN-10: 0-471-43030-7 • $14.95

KEEP YOUR BRAIN YOUNG:
The Complete Guide to Physical and Emotional Health and Longevity

Guy M. McKhann, M.D., and Marilyn Albert, Ph.D.

Every aspect of aging and the brain: changes in memory, nutrition, mood, sleep, and sex, as well as the later problems in alcohol use, vision, hearing, movement, and balance.

Cloth • 304 pp • ISBN-10: 0-471-40792-5 • $24.95
Paper • 304 pp • ISBN-10: 0-471-43028-5 • $15.95

THE END OF STRESS AS WE KNOW IT

Bruce S. McEwen, Ph.D., with Elizabeth Norton Lasley • *Foreword by Robert Sapolsky*

How brain and body work under stress and how it is possible to avoid its debilitating effects.

Cloth • 239 pp • ISBN-10: 0-309-07640-4 • $27.95
Paper • 262 pp • ISBN-10: 0-309-09121-7 • $19.95

IN SEARCH OF THE LOST CORD:
Solving the Mystery of Spinal Cord Regeneration

Luba Vikhanski

The story of the scientists and science involved in the international scientific race to find ways to repair the damaged spinal cord and restore movement.

21 photos; 12 illustrations.

Cloth • 269 pp • ISBN-10: 0-309-07437-1 • $27.95

THE SECRET LIFE OF THE BRAIN

Richard Restak, M.D. • *Foreword by David Grubin*

Companion book to the PBS series of the same name, exploring recent discoveries about the brain from infancy through old age.

Cloth • 201 pp • ISBN-10: 0-309-07435-5 • $35.00

THE LONGEVITY STRATEGY:
How to Live to 100 Using the Brain-Body Connection

David Mahoney and Richard Restak, M.D. • *Foreword by William Safire*

Advice on the brain and aging well.

Cloth • 250 pp • ISBN-10: 0-471-24867-3 • $22.95
Paper • 272 pp • ISBN-10: 0-471-32794-8 • $14.95

STATES OF MIND:
New Discoveries About How Our Brains Make Us Who We Are

Roberta Conlan, Editor

Adapted from the Dana/Smithsonian Associates lecture series by eight of the country's top brain scientists, including the 2000 Nobel laureate in medicine, Eric Kandel.

Cloth • 214 pp • ISBN-10: 0-471-29963-4 • $24.95
Paper • 224 pp • ISBN-10: 0-471-39973-6 • $18.95

The Dana Foundation Series on Neuroethics

DEFINING RIGHT AND WRONG IN BRAIN SCIENCE:
Essential Readings in Neuroethics

Walter Glannon, Ph.D., Editor

The fifth volume in The Dana Foundation Series on Neuroethics, this collection marks the five-year anniversary of the first meeting in the field of neuroethics, providing readers with the seminal writings on the past, present, and future ethical issues facing neuroscience and society.

Cloth • 350 pp • ISBN-10: 978-1-932594-25-6 • $15.95

HARD SCIENCE, HARD CHOICES:
Facts, Ethics, and Policies Guiding Brain Science Today

Sandra J. Ackerman, Editor

Top scholars and scientists discuss new and complex medical and social ethics brought about by advances in neuroscience. Based on an invitational meeting co-sponsored by the Library of Congress, the National Institutes of Health, the Columbia University Center for Bioethics, and the Dana Foundation.

Paper • 152 pp • ISBN-10: 1-932594-02-7 • $12.95

NEUROSCIENCE AND THE LAW: Brain, Mind, and the Scales of Justice

Brent Garland, Editor. With commissioned papers by Michael S. Gazzaniga, Ph.D., and Megan S. Steven; Laurence R. Tancredi, M.D., J.D.; Henry T. Greely, J.D.; and Stephen J. Morse, J.D., Ph.D.

How discoveries in neuroscience influence criminal and civil justice, based on an invitational meeting of 26 top neuroscientists, legal scholars, attorneys, and state and federal judges convened by the Dana Foundation and the American Association for the Advancement of Science.

Paper • 226 pp • ISBN-10: 1-032594-04-3 • $8.95

BEYOND THERAPY: Biotechnology and the Pursuit of Happiness
A Report of the President's Council on Bioethics

Special Foreword by Leon R. Kass, M.D., Chairman

Introduction by William Safire

Can biotechnology satisfy human desires for better children, superior performance, ageless bodies, and happy souls? This report says these possibilities present us with profound ethical challenges and choices. Includes dissenting commentary by scientist members of the Council.

Paper • 376 pp • ISBN-10: 1-932594-05-1 • $10.95

NEUROETHICS: Mapping the Field. Conference Proceedings

Steven J. Marcus, Editor

Proceedings of the landmark 2002 conference organized by Stanford University and the University of California, San Francisco, and sponsored by the Dana Foundation, at which more than 150 neuroscientists, bioethicists, psychiatrists and psychologists, philosophers, and professors of law and public policy debated the ethical implications of neuroscience research findings.

50 illustrations.

Paper • 367 pp • ISBN-10: 0-9723830-0-X • $10.95

Immunology

RESISTANCE: The Human Struggle Against Infection

Norbert Gualde, M.D., translated by Steven Rendall

Traces the histories of epidemics and the emergence or re-emergence of diseases, illustrating how new global strategies and research of the body's own weapons of immunity can work together to fight tomorrow's inevitable infectious outbreaks.

Cloth • 219 pp • ISBN-10: 1-932594-00-0 • $25.00

FATAL SEQUENCE: The Killer Within

Kevin J. Tracey, M.D.

An easily understood account of the spiral of sepsis, a sometimes fatal crisis that most often affects patients fighting off nonfatal illnesses or injury. Tracey puts the scientific and medical story of sepsis in the context of his battle to save a burned baby, a sensitive telling of cutting-edge science.

Cloth • 231 pp • ISBN-10: 1-932594-06-X • $23.95
Paper • 231 pp • ISBN-10: 1-932594-09-4 • $12.95

Arts Education

A WELL-TEMPERED MIND: Using Music to Help Children Listen and Learn

Peter Perret and Janet Fox • Foreword by Maya Angelou

Five musicians enter elementary school classrooms, helping children learn about music and contributing to both higher enthusiasm and improved academic performance. This charming story gives us a taste of things to come in one of the newest areas of brain research: the effect of music on the brain.

12 illustrations.

Cloth • 225 pp • ISBN-10: 1-932594-03-5 • $22.95
Paper • 225 pp • ISBN-10: 1-932594-08-6 • $12.00

Dana Press also publishes periodicals dealing with brain science, arts education, and immunology. For more information, visit www.dana.org.